HANDBOOK OF
PSYCHIATRIC
EMERGENCIES

HANDBOOK <u>OF</u>
PSYCHIATRIC
EMERGENCIES

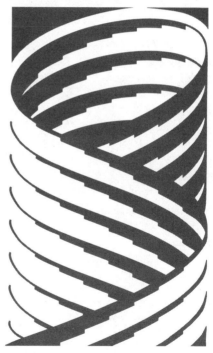

William R. Dubin, MD
Kenneth J. Weiss, MD

Springhouse Corporation
Springhouse, Pennsylvania

STAFF

Executive Director, Editorial
Stanley Loeb

Director of Trade and Textbooks
Minnie B. Rose, RN, BSN, MEd

Art Director
John Hubbard

Senior Acquisitions Editor
Susan L. Mease

Editors
David Moreau, Karen Zimmermann

Copy Editor
Mary Hohenhaus Hardy

Designers
Stephanie Peters (associate art director), Lesley Weissman-Cook

Art Production
Robert Perry (manager), Anna Brindisi, Donald Knauss, Tom Robbins, Robert Wieder

Typography
David Kosten (director), Diane Paluba (manager), Elizabeth Bergman, Joyce Rossi Biletz, Phyllis Marron, Robin Rantz, Valerie Rosenberger

Manufacturing
Deborah Meiris (manager), T.A. Landis, Jennifer Suter

Production Coordination
Colleen M. Hayman

Library of Congress Cataloging-in-Publication Data

Dubin, William R.
  Handbook of psychiatric emergencies/William R. Dubin, Kenneth J. Weiss.
     p. cm.
  Includes bibliographical references and index.
  1. Psychiatric emergencies—Handbooks, manuals, etc. 2. Psychiatric nursing—Handbooks, manuals, etc. I. Weiss, Kenneth J. II. Title.
  [DNLM: 1. Emergency Services, Psychiatric—handbooks. WM 34 D814h]
RC480.6.D82   1991
616.89′025—dc20
DNLM/DLC   90-10424
ISBN 0-87434-330-5   CIP

CONTENTS

CONTRIBUTORS

William R. Dubin, MD
Deputy Medical Director
Philadelphia Psychiatric Center
Professor of Psychiatry
Temple University School of Medicine, Philadelphia

Kenneth J. Weiss, MD
Head, Division of Ambulatory Care and Director, Psychiatric
    Residency Training
Cooper Hospital/University Medical Center
Professor of Clinical Psychiatry
University of Medicine and Dentistry of New Jersey
Robert Wood Johnson Medical School, Camden

Howard Dichter, MD
Director, Family Therapy and Director, Comprehensive Treatment
    Center
Philadelphia Psychiatric Center
Clinical Assistant Professor
Temple University School of Medicine, Philadelphia
(Chapter 11)

Gail Greenspan, MD
Clinical Assistant Professor of Psychiatry
Assistant Director, Jefferson Psychiatric Associates
Jefferson Medical College, Philadelphia
(Chapter 12)

Susan M. Ice
Director, Adolescent Unit and Eating Disorders Programs
Philadelphia Psychiatric Center
Assistant Clinical Professor of Psychiatry
Temple University School of Medicine, Philadelphia
(Chapter 13)

Sherry Carroll Pomerantz, PhD
Research Psychologist
Albert Einstein Medical Center, Philadelphia
(Chapter 11)

ACKNOWLEDGMENTS

We would like to thank our parents, Bernice and Bill Weiss and Sidney and Sylvia Dubin, without whom none of this would have been possible; Elizabeth Kramer, whose energy provided us with the initial impetus to write this book; our chairmen, Drs. Paul Fink and Harvey Strassman, who provided the atmosphere and encouragement that allowed us to complete the book; and Marie Horn and Barbara Pauly for their tireless help in typing the many drafts.

DEDICATION
This book is dedicated with love and affection to our wives, Alicia and Susan, and our children, Brian, Aaron, and Naomi.

PREFACE

Most psychiatric emergencies are treated by nonpsychiatrists in a service located in or adjacent to the emergency department of a general hospital, yet psychiatric literature specifically tailored for the nonspecialist is surprisingly scarce. *Handbook of Psychiatric Emergencies* was written for the nonpsychiatrist to supplement direct clinical supervision. The book is not meant to be a comprehensive reference on psychiatry or psychiatric emergencies, but rather a concise, practical guide to what nonpsychiatrists or first-year psychiatric residents need to know to manage a psychiatric emergency for a few hours without the assistance of an experienced psychiatrist.

Treatment of any psychiatric emergency involves three primary tasks. The first is to rule out medical illness as a cause of the emergency. When appropriate, we present the medical evaluation and highlight the possible underlying medical causes. Failure to appreciate the role of physical illness in precipitating a psychiatric emergency can have devastating consequences. The second task is to reduce the risk that the patient will harm himself or others; the third, to determine the best treatment setting for the patient: inpatient, outpatient, day hospital, or crisis intervention. Establishing a final diagnosis and initiating a definitive treatment are usually not emergency intervention goals. Instead, the emergency services clinician treats syndromes, such as psychosis, violent behavior, or suicidal ideation.

Consequently, each chapter addresses a series of questions from the perspective of an emergency services clinician: "What are the patient's symptoms? What might be the cause? What is the best intervention?" Chapter 1 explains how to prepare for the patient interview (planning an appropriate setting, anticipating the patient's needs, reviewing the elements to document on the clinical record) and how to conduct a thorough mental status examination (assessing the patient's behavior, thought, emotions, perceptual disturbances, orientation, and intellect).

Chapter 2 focuses on important medicolegal issues that might arise from contact with the patient: confidentiality, documentation, competence and informed consent, civil commitment, the clinician's duty to warn and protect a violent patient's potential victims, liability, and patients' rights.

Chapters 3 to 14 cover the most prevalent psychiatric conditions encountered by clinicians in the emergency setting: delirium, alcohol and drug emergencies, schizophrenia and mania, violent and self-destructive behavior, depression, anxiety, domestic abuse, rape, child and adolescent emergencies, and geriatric emergencies.

Chapter 15 reviews various situations that can prove especially frustrating for the clinician, including patients who feign illness to obtain drugs, attention, or temporary shelter; callers who abuse telephone hotlines; language barriers presented by non-English-speaking patients; and disposition difficulties when trying to place patients in hospitals or other agencies.

Chapter 16 highlights appropriate treatment interventions for patients who are experiencing unwanted side effects from antipsychotics, antidepressants, lithium carbonate, antianxiety drugs, anticonvulsants, antihistamines, beta blockers, or disulfiram.

Where appropriate, information is organized under recurring headings to help the user identify the problem, intervene safely and effectively, and complete the disposition of the patient. *Identifying the problem* presents information to distinguish the patient's condition from others that may mimic it; thus, the section reviews mental status findings, physical findings, laboratory studies, and differential diagnoses. *Interpersonal intervention* examines what to say and do during the interview to make the patient feel more comfortable, promote more effective communication, and minimize or possibly resolve the crisis. *Pharmacologic intervention* focuses on drug treatments that may prove effective in reducing symptoms when interpersonal interventions fail to resolve the emergency. *Educational intervention* outlines relevant issues to discuss with the patient and family, such as teaching them to recognize early signs and symptoms of a problem, explaining preventive measures they can take to thwart or minimize a recurrence, and informing them of appropriate community resources that can provide additional help. *Disposition* examines options in handling the patient's case – discharge, hospitalization, consultation, or referral – depending on his physical, psychiatric, and socioeconomic needs. Finally, *Medicolegal considerations* summarizes the legal principles that are relevant to the problem being discussed.

References at the end of each chapter provide an excellent source for further investigation of topics, and four appendices — signs and symptoms of major psychiatric syndromes, a decision tree for psychosis, a mini-mental state examination, and a glossary of street drug names — serve as handy, helpful resources for quick reference.

Managing psychiatric emergencies can be a stressful, complicated, and frustrating responsibility, especially for the nonpsychiatrist. The keys to successfully treating patients with various psychiatric problems are sufficient knowledge of psychiatric syndromes and sufficient confidence to develop diagnostic, interpersonal, and patient-teaching skills. Toward that end, we hope this handbook proves to be an invaluable source of information and encouragement.

William R. Dubin, MD
Kenneth J. Weiss, MD

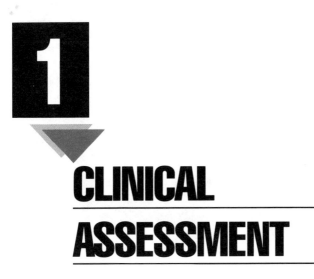

CLINICAL
ASSESSMENT

This chapter provides the clinician with the basic tools for evaluating patients with psychiatric complaints. It outlines the essential clinical assessment—the mental status examination—and describes necessary preparation. Using the tools discussed in the following pages, you will be prepared to work effectively with the wide variety of patients described in later chapters.

PATIENT PRESENTATION

You may encounter a patient with psychiatric complaints in many different situations. For example, a patient may require help because of mental discomfort—sadness, agitation, or drug side effects. A family member or caregiver may request an evaluation for a child with wild behavior, an elderly parent who wanders, or a paranoid patient who threatens others in a community-living arrangement. Psychiatric evaluation may be necessary because of a disruptive event—rape, child abuse, or an automobile or industrial accident. A person who has inflicted self-harm, either a suicide gesture or attempt, is in need of psychiatric care. An intoxicated person may ask for help over the telephone, or the police may bring in a hallucinating or threatening person.

In preparing to render service in an emergency, try to develop a sense of the severity of the patient's complaints, based on his behavior. Perform as complete an assessment as the situation allows. Walker (1983) lists three groups into which psychiatric patients can be categorized:

Emergency
- Impending or active alcohol withdrawal syndrome
- Violent behavior
- Drug toxicity
- Suicide attempts

Urgency
- Bizarre behavior
- Acute agitation
- Suicidal or homicidal risk
- Inebriation
- Evaluations for civil commitment
- Suicide gestures

Nonemergency
- Situational disturbances (marital discord, family disturbance, poverty)
- Mild to moderate anxiety
- Desire "to talk"
- Medication questions, refills, side effects
- Known patients needing support

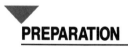

PREPARATION

Preparation for any psychiatric examination should include plans for creating an appropriate environment, anticipating your initial response to the emergency and the outcome of the visit, and reviewing pertinent data that you must document in the clinical record.

Appropriate environment

The clinician preparing to examine a psychiatric patient should take the time to create the best environment. Before examining any patient, you may want to consider these factors:

▪ **Space.** Privacy, reasonable physical comfort, and minimal noise and lighting help reduce patient stimulation. If necessary, you may have to examine a wildly delirious patient who is restrained on a stretcher, but whenever possible, move the patient to the most soothing surroundings available.

▪ **Support.** Maximize clinician-patient interaction by providing a supportive environment (for example, by attending to the patient's need for food and drink, toileting, and attention from caring persons).

▪ **Security.** If you consider the patient dangerous, security (ranging from observation to physical restraint) must precede clinical work. The session will ultimately be more productive if you and the patient feel safe.

▪ **Family and friends.** Unless the patient insists on privacy, query any available family members or friends to help fill in details, add perspective, or directly resolve conflicts. Never overlook an opportunity to broaden the clinical data base.

▪ **Time.** Few clinicians have the luxury of treating one patient at a time, from start to finish. Rather, several situations of varying acuity typically demand attention. As early as possible, assess the time needed to address a particular problem. For example, a serious overdose case may take only a few minutes to determine that the patient needs to be admitted for treatment, whereas a marital dispute with a threat of violence may require a 2-hour initial session and perhaps follow-up visits.

▪ **Objectives.** Always remember your ultimate goal—to return the patient to his previous level of functioning or to refer him to a facility for special care—and try to help the patient understand this goal as early as possible so that he does not develop false expectations of the outcome. Interventions in a psychiatric emergency, important but modest in scope, include ruling out medical illness, stabilizing the patient, and determining the most appropriate treatment setting—inpatient, outpatient, partial (day) hospital, or residential.

Initial response

Your first task is to decide how quickly the patient should be seen and whether security precautions are needed to ensure patient and staff safety. Before addressing such details as diagnosis and drug dosages, determine the overall clinical perspective by asking these questions:

• What were the circumstances surrounding the request for treatment? Is the patient present voluntarily or involuntarily?

• Do any staff clinicians know the patient? Can they provide reliable information about the course and outcome of previous visits?

• Are records from previous visits accessible?

• Does a social support system exist? How readily can it be mobilized?

• Have family members or friends accompanied the patient? Can they provide a reliable patient history?

Anticipation of outcome

As complicated as psychiatric problems may seem to be, a psychiatric emergency visit can result in only four potential outcomes: obtaining a psychiatric consultation, referring the patient to a nonpsychiatric physician for further evaluation and treatment, admitting the patient to the hospital, or discharging him with a referral to a mental health or social service provider (Walker, 1983). Keep these outcomes in mind during your evaluation, and remember that some patients will leave the emergency setting before evaluation or treatment can begin. Only those patients assessed as dangerous can be legally detained against their will.

Clinical record

Ideally, the permanent record of your contact with a patient should include the following:

▪ **Chief complaint.** Indicate why the patient is seeking treatment. Use direct quotations from the patient, such as "I drank too much."

▪ **Identifying data.** Record the patient's age, sex, marital status, occupation, and residence, and note whether the patient is known to the emergency staff.

▪ **History of the problem.** Comment on the problem in terms of the patient's recent status, as in "Patient was in his usual state of health until [time], when [event]." Then briefly describe how the event led to this visit.

■ **Psychiatric history.** What past or current contacts has the person had with the mental health system? Who is the current health care provider? Is the patient on medication? If so, which, how much, and how often? Explore medication compliance.

■ **Medical history.** Which conditions or treatments might help explain the current problem?

■ **Mental status examination.** Which observable features lead to a diagnosis?

■ **Physical examination.** Do any signs lead to a diagnosis of an organic mental disorder?

■ **Diagnostic tests.** How can the clinical laboratory help distinguish among differential diagnoses?

■ **Family and friends.** What can others reveal about the patient's behavior?

■ **Diagnosis.** Is the patient suffering from an organic disorder (such as delirium), a psychosis (such as mania), or an adjustment disorder (such as transitory depression)? For those unfamiliar with psychiatric diagnosis, the *Diagnostic and Statistical Manual of the American Psychiatric Association,* 3rd edition, revised *(DSM-III-R)* is a valuable resource that should be available in the emergency service.

■ **Treatment provided.** Document all interpersonal, medical, and social interventions thoroughly. Include all personal or telephone contacts with family and friends, physicians, therapists, and others. For medication, include the time, dosage, desired effects, side effects, and patient-teaching instructions given.

■ **Disposition.** Record clearly how the diagnosis was made, especially when discharging a violent or self-destructive patient, because the last clinician to treat a patient can be held liable if the patient subsequently harms himself or others.

▼
MENTAL STATUS EXAMINATION

Assessing and documenting the patient's mental status is the core of any emergency intervention (see the Appendices for quick-reference charts that can be helpful in performing a thorough mental status examination). A carefully conducted mental status examination is important because it:

• provides a basis for diagnosis, especially to differentiate organic from functional disorders
• identifies target signs or symptoms for treatment
• documents what was or was not observed
• serves as a useful record for future comparison.

The mental status examination can uncover a mental disorder in the same way that a physical examination can reveal an organic disorder. Structural elements of the examination include the patient's behavior, thought, emotions, percepts (perceptual disturbances), orientation, and intellect (cognitive function).

Behavior

Within the first few minutes of contact with a patient, begin to collect clinical data based on the following categories:

■ **Appearance.** Attire and personal grooming reflect the patient's ability to care for himself and make appropriate judgments. If the patient is neat and well groomed, psychosis is an unlikely diagnosis. However, a disheveled and unkempt appearance can suggest schizophrenia, depression, substance abuse, or dementia. A bizarre and eccentric appearance suggests schizophrenia or mania; a careless or indifferent appearance suggests depression or substance abuse.

■ **Movement.** The patient's motor behavior also can provide data that will aid in diagnosis. For example, fine and coarse tremors or pill-rolling finger movements can indicate anxiety, alcohol withdrawal, or neuroleptic-induced parkinsonism. Agitation (pacing, restlessness, generalized motor excitement) suggests mania, schizophrenia, anxiety, stimulant use, or drug or alcohol withdrawal. Motor retardation (slow initiation of movement) could signal catatonia, depression, or parkinsonism. Extrapyramidal symptoms, such as akathisia (motor restlessness), akinesia (absence of movement), and dyskinesia (grimacing or writhing movements), may be signs of antipsychotic drug side effects.

■ **Speech.** Measure the patient's verbal ability in terms of spontaneity, pressure, rate, tone, volume, and articulation. Speech patterns can be a valuable indicator of the patient's mental status. Mutism usually suggests schizophrenia or depression. Slow speech could signal depression. Rapid, uninterrupted speech suggests mania, extreme anxiety, or stimulant use, whereas slurred speech probably means that the patient is intoxicated. Dementia is a likely diagnosis if the patient is aphasic (can no longer express or comprehend spoken or written language). An unusual use of words suggests schizophrenia or organic mental disorder. Examples include *neologism* (new word created by, and having special meaning for, the patient), *word salad* (incoherent mixture of words and phrases), *echolalia* (repetition of another person's words), and *perseveration* (repetition of a word, phrase, or idea in response to varied stimuli).

Thought

A person's thought should be goal directed, coherent, and responsive to outside stimuli. Thought patterns that do not meet these criteria may indicate psychosis. *Circumstantiality,* the thought pattern of a patient who reaches a goal after numerous unnecessary digressions, suggests schizophrenia, organic mental disorder, or obsessive-compulsive disorder. In contrast, *tangentiality,* a thought pattern that veers off the subject and does not return, suggests schizophrenia only. Manic patients typically exhibit a *flight of ideas,* a rapid succession of context-bound and comprehensible thoughts. On the other hand, schizophrenic patients may demonstrate a *looseness of association* (also called *derailment*), a succession of irrelevant and usually incomprehensible thoughts.

Thought content also can provide insight into a patient's mental status. A careful assessment of thought content may reveal that a patient is delusional, obsessive-compulsive, or suicidal. A *delusion* is a fixed, false belief not shared by other members of the patient's culture or subculture. The patient maintains this belief despite all evidence against it. Delusions of persecution or grandeur suggest schizophrenia, mania, or stimulant intoxication. Delusions involving religious ideas (for example, "I am God" or "God has given me special powers") could be signs of schizophrenia or mania. Delusions of guilt, poverty, or disease may reflect psychotic depression. A patient who has delusions of a partner's infidelity may be suffering from a paranoid disorder. Inquire about the content of the delusions, and gently discover if they can be modified by logic; for example, "Is it possible that your house is not bugged?" Do not directly challenge a patient's delusional ideas; this may cause a rift in the patient-clinician relationship.

Ideas of reference (marked by a belief that people are talking about or referring to the patient by means of gestures or expressions) suggest schizophrenia or chronic stimulant abuse. Ask the patient, "When you see two people talking to each other but can't hear them, do you think they are talking about you?"

A patient with an *obsession* feels compelled to have unwanted, intrusive thoughts, sometimes accompanied by compulsive behavior. For example, a patient may exhibit an obsessional idea of contamination coupled with a handwashing compulsion. Such behavior suggests obsessive-compulsive disorder, which is an anxiety disorder rather than a psychosis. To assess for obsessive thought, ask the patient, "Do you ever have an idea that you can't get out of your head?"

Suicidal thoughts, including a preoccupation with the method to use, suggest depression, personality disorder, or any mental disorder accompanied by a depressed mood (such as alcoholism or psychosis). To elicit thoughts of suicide, ask the patient, "Do you ever feel that life is not worth living? Are you planning to take your life? Do you have the means to do it?" A mental status examination is incomplete if the examiner fails to document whether or not the patient has had suicidal thoughts.

Homicidal thoughts suggest psychosis or personality disorder. Such thoughts manifest themselves as a preoccupation with killing someone, not always a specific victim. Ask the patient, "Do you ever feel like hurting someone? How close are you to doing it? Do you own weapons or have other means to do it? Have you ever been arrested, and if so, for what?"

Emotions

A sustained emotion is called a *mood.* Although moods cannot be observed directly, an examiner can determine the patient's emotional tone — happy, sad, angry, frightened — by asking, "What were you feeling that made you come here today?"

An *affect* is a short-lived emotional expression of a mood that can be observed by the examiner, who must determine whether the affect matches the patient's reported mood and is appropriate to the content of the thought. An inappropriate affect does not fit the situation; for example, laughing about a sad event. Inappropriate emotions suggest schizophrenia or milder forms of anxiety. A flat (blunted) affect, characterized by expressionless speech and facial appearance regardless of the situation, may suggest schizophrenia or neuroleptic-induced parkinsonism. A labile affect, characterized by unstable, rapidly changing emotions, may be a sign of dementia, mania, or intoxication. Euphoric affects — expansive emotional expressions not justified by the circumstances — suggest mania or stimulant abuse.

Percepts

A disturbance in perception occurs when the patient has difficulty distinguishing between sensory stimulation and inner feelings (Hanke, 1984). Perceptual disturbances include illusions and hallucinations.

An *illusion* is a false interpretation of real events, commonly under conditions of low levels of auditory or visual stimulation. During the interview, ask the patient, "Does your mind ever play tricks on you?" Although some illusions are normal, they can also occur in drug abuse disorders and paranoia.

A *hallucination* is a sensory perception without sensory input: the patient perceives something that is not there. Auditory hallucinations, the most common type, suggest schizophrenia or alcoholic hallucinosis. Other types of hallucinations are visual (suggesting delirium, alcohol or drug withdrawal, or drug intoxication), tactile (suggesting delirium or chronic stimulant abuse), and olfactory or gustatory (suggesting epilepsy).

Orientation and intellect

Patient orientation and cognitive function can help you distinguish between organic and other mental disorders. Defects in one or more of the following areas suggest delirium, dementia, or drug-induced conditions:

▪ **Orientation.** A person's orientation is easily lost for time, sometimes for place, but rarely for who he is. Suspect malingering (feigning illness for some concrete benefit) if a patient tells you, in clear consciousness, that he doesn't know his name.

▪ **Memory.** A person's ability to recall is influenced by intelligence, age, and mood, such as depression or anxiety. A patient with dementia usually has trouble with recent memory, whereas a patient with delirium has more global deficits. Useful questions to test memory include: "Who is the President? What is happening in the world? What are the names and ages of your children?"

■ **Attention and concentration.** The patient's ability to sustain a cognitive effort can be determined by having him subtract by sevens from 100.

■ **Calculation.** The patient's ability to perform calculations should be measured against his level of education. For example, an accountant who cannot do simple arithmetic may have a profound deficit.

■ **Abstraction.** A person's ability to think in abstract terms is influenced by education and intelligence. One test of abstraction is whether the patient can describe the similarities between two things, such as a dog and a cat or an apple and a banana. Proverb interpretation (for instance, asking the patient to explain the figurative meaning of "Look before you leap" or "Don't cry over spilled milk") can test both abstraction ability and thought content.

■ **Judgment and insight.** How a patient assesses a situation can help you determine whether he needs in-hospital treatment. Sound *judgment* depends on intact consciousness, orientation, memory, attention, and concentration and can be assessed by asking the patient about a real or imaginary situation. For example, ask the patient, "What do you think should be done about this problem?" *Insight* reflects the patient's awareness of a psychological problem, although not necessarily its cause. Patients with psychoses and organic mental disorders usually lack insight, which can be assessed by asking, "What do you think the problem is?"

REFERENCES

Hanke, N. *Handbook of Emergency Psychiatry.* Lexington, Mass.: Collamore Press, 1984.

Walker, J.I. *Psychiatric Emergencies: Intervention and Resolution.* Philadelphia: J.B. Lippincott Co., 1983.

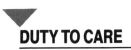

2

MEDICOLEGAL
CONSIDERATIONS

Before attempting any psychiatric interventions, the clinician must understand the fundamentals of emergency psychiatry, one of which is knowing the relationship between psychiatry and the law. This chapter addresses medicolegal questions that typically arise for the nonspecialist ("Do I have to see this patient? How can I communicate with others about a patient without revealing confidential information? What do I do with a dangerous patient? How do I avoid getting sued?") and explains why you cannot afford to ignore legal issues in your practice.

DUTY TO CARE

People create, modify, and break various kinds of agreements and obligations, some informal, such as keeping an appointment, and some formal, such as a contract for goods or services. By law, the clinician-patient relationship, once established, is an agreement between the two parties that creates for the clinician an obligation or duty to provide the patient with needed care. This does not mean that a clinician in an office setting must care for every patient requesting service, and no health care professional should provide a service for which he has no training.

The situation in a psychiatric emergency service is somewhat different from that in an office setting. In the emergency service, the duty to care is created automatically, by virtue of the service's existence. And because the clinician has no sure way of immediately discriminating between an emergency and a nonemergency, all patients must be treated as if an emergency—and thus the duty to care—existed. For example, a duty to care is automatically created when:

• a patient enters a hospital emergency department and asks to see a psychiatrist or a counselor
• a person calls an established hotline to discuss suicidal feelings
• a patient who usually rejects psychiatric help asks to be seen
• the police bring a person into the emergency department
• an outreach service is asked to see a disturbed person in the community.

Thus, if you work in any setting that provides emergency psychiatric services, the answer to the question "Do I have to see this patient?" is an unqualified "Yes!" And keep in mind that fulfilling the duty to care does not protect you against future allegations of professional misconduct. Clinicians must fulfill other duties, such as the duty to treat the patient according to the standards of care established in the community and the duty to protect the patient and others from the patient's behavior.

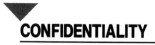

CONFIDENTIALITY

Because the clinician-patient relationship is built on trust, the confidential nature of information provided by the patient is one of the cornerstones of practice. Breaking that trust would undermine the therapeutic alliance and seriously impede therapy (Simon, 1986). Confidentiality in the practice of emergency psychiatry is based on the following:

■ **Tradition.** Patients expect that what they say will be kept confidential.

- **Statute.** Most states have laws that require health care professionals to maintain patient confidentiality, with specified penalties for failing to do so.
- **Ethics.** The Oath of Hippocrates, the American Medical Association, and the American Psychiatric Association explicitly prohibit breach of confidentiality, except in specific circumstances. Similar constraints apply to nurses, mental health workers, social workers, and psychologists.
- **Case law.** Physicians and other health care professionals have been held liable for harm done to patients because of a breach of confidentiality (Simon, 1986). Breach of this duty is considered a tort, or civil wrong, and is grounds for a lawsuit.

Be aware that the duty to maintain confidentiality gives way to a higher duty — preserving the health and welfare of the patient and others — in certain situations. For instance, you may need to reveal confidential information to prevent a suicidal or homicidal patient from causing harm; to consult with other clinicians about a patient who needs emergency treatment, especially if the patient cannot or will not talk to you about his condition; to protect a defenseless person, such as an abused child, from further harm; or to present clinical information about a patient in a court hearing to determine whether the patient should be committed to a mental institution. You also can reveal confidential information if a patient consents to the revelation or if the patient is a minor and you must discuss his condition with a parent or legal guardian.

Although a psychiatric emergency may necessitate a breach of confidentiality, the patient does not lose his right to privacy. Unnecessary personal details should not be included in the medical record. The *law of parsimony* applies to all disclosures; that is, the clinician should disclose the least amount of confidential information needed for evaluation, treatment, or disposition. If any information must be disclosed to others, the patient should be informed whenever possible and any requests to maintain privacy should be honored, as long as the patient's health is not compromised.

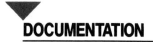

DOCUMENTATION

The clinical record documents what was done and why it was done. Documentation in the emergency setting should be sufficiently comprehensive to form a permanent record of the patient's complaint, interventions taken by the clinician, and disposition; to be informative to other professionals who may be using the record as a basis for future clinical decisions; and to satisfy third parties, such as insurance companies, lawyers, and courts, about the nature and quality of the psychiatric evaluation. The clinical record should also indicate whether the service rendered was within the required standard of care. This includes satisfying any third party that other legal duties were fulfilled, such as the duty to call a child protection agency if you suspect child abuse or the duty to warn a person whom a patient has threatened.

For the reasons noted above – and because the clinical record can serve as evidence in court proceedings – documentation should be complete and accurate. Follow these guidelines when completing the record of any patient you see in an emergency setting:

• Note how the clinical contact was established. Did the patient come independently, or was he sent by an agency or brought by police?

• In defining the chief complaint, indicate what made the visit an emergency in the patient's mind. Document the complaint by quoting the patient directly.

• In recording results of the mental status examination, mention whether you assessed danger to the patient or others, including whether the patient possessed the means to carry out a threat and any history of self-destructive or violent behavior.

• Be sure to include clinical reasoning in your documentation. If a patient has fully recovered from a drug overdose and you rule out a suicide attempt, make sure the record reflects your justification for discharging the patient.

• For any patient who refuses treatment, note whether he was mentally competent to understand the consequences of refusal. Failure to treat an incompetent patient who refuses may be considered negligent (Simon, 1986).

• Note all follow-up instructions given to the patient. Many emergency centers use multicopy forms, one of which is given to the patient on discharge and another that is retained in the patient's permanent record.

• Avoid slang, jargon, or pejorative labels. Assume that the record will be read later by the patient and his lawyer.

• Document all interventions thoroughly. From a legal standpoint, any intervention not included in the record did not occur. Remembering that you had tried to dissuade a suicide victim from his intentions will not carry much legal weight if you fail to include this in your notes and the victim's family subsequently sues you for failure to prevent the death.

COMPETENCE AND CONSENT

Under the law, all adults are presumed to be competent (able to make decisions about important matters) unless judged by a court to be incompetent. In a psychiatric emergency, however, waiting for a court to act is rarely feasible; therefore, the patient's ability to make decisions is based on *clinical competence.* A patient's clinical competence becomes a factor when he consents to or refuses treatment or hospitalization. An assessment of clinical competence may be warranted, for instance, when a psychotic or dangerous patient refuses treatment or when consent for treatment cannot be obtained. The main criteria used by clinicians to assess a patient's clinical competence are orientation to time, place, and person; awareness of the psychological condition under consideration; understanding of the potential benefits and risks of a proposed treatment; and understanding of the consequences of refusing treatment.

Clinical implications of competence

A patient who is delirious, grossly psychotic, demented, or intoxicated is probably not competent to make decisions. In such cases, try to obtain consent for treatment from family members. If the patient is dangerous, consent issues are less important, because most state laws permit treatment of a dangerous patient against his will. If alternate consent is unavailable, you can, in good faith, treat a severely psychotic patient; indeed, failure to do so could be considered negligent.

Definition of consent

Informed consent has become a standard consideration in medical and nursing practice. The three basic elements of consent are information, competence, and voluntariness (Simon, 1986).

Information. A patient cannot be expected to consent to or refuse treatment without having enough information to weigh the risks and benefits. The clinician is responsible for providing this information, including whatever the patient might want to know about treatment side effects, legally known as *material risk*. To satisfy the legal requirements for informed consent, you cannot merely recite a list of side effects. Rather, discuss all treatment side effects that could reasonably make a difference to the patient about whether to accept or reject treatment. Furthermore, you cannot withhold treatment information for fear that the patient will refuse treatment based on the information.

Competence. Many mentally retarded, psychotic, and organically impaired patients are not clinically competent to understand treatment information or to make a decision. In such cases, try to obtain consent from a family member. In a true emergency, competence is of secondary concern.

Voluntariness. Consent to treatment must be given voluntarily; that is, with free will. The clinical concept of free will – the absence of being forced to choose – is practical rather than philosophical. To say "Sign this admission paper or I will call the police" is a type of coercion that negates voluntariness. Any treatment given under conditions of a threat could be seen by a court as assault and battery.

You must obtain consent before beginning any intervention for a child, including parental consent for any child younger than age 16 and additional consent from adolescents, beginning at approximately age 14. An adolescent who is legally emancipated and competent can sign for procedures. Additionally, you should honor an adolescent's request for confidentiality unless the adolescent poses a danger to himself or others or you suspect child abuse. Because the formal age of consent varies from state to state, each clinical service should have written policies and procedures governing these situations.

Consent in practice

Informed consent procedures should become an automatic part of every clinical interaction. When possible, the patient should sign a written consent form. Some states require written informed consent for each psychotropic drug administered. At a minimum, document that you discussed proposed benefits and potential risks of treatment with the patient. Consent should not be set aside except under conditions of manifest danger to the patient or others. Even then, when the emergency subsides, the patient usually retains the right to refuse treatment and to be supplied with information about potential risks.

Scenario for clinical evaluation

To ensure that all patients are assessed for competence and that they are provided with sufficient information to give an informed consent, cover the following points during the initial examination:
• Assess the patient's orientation to time, place, and person. What is the patient's understanding of the emergency visit?
• Inform the patient of your role, your understanding of the clinical situation, and how you propose to assess the need for treatment.
• Explain your clinical findings, what they mean, and what can be done to remedy the situation (including crisis intervention, medication, or hospitalization).
• Have the patient reiterate, in his own words, your explanation of the situation, and then solicit his questions or comments.
• Explain the treatment's potential side effects.
• Ask specific questions to determine whether the patient understands the benefits and risks of treatment.
• Obtain written consent from the patient, if possible.

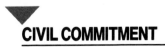

CIVIL COMMITMENT

Traditionally, governments have had a legal right to take charge of a citizen in the best interests of society. Thus, all states have civil commitment statutes that permit detention of mentally ill persons under certain circumstances. Nonpsychiatrists must be familiar with state commitment laws because some patients must be detained while awaiting a psychiatric evaluation or legal adjudication.

Inform the patient if you're considering commitment, and never use commitment as a weapon or threat. Instead, say, "We have determined that we must hospitalize you for your mental problem so that everyone is safe. We are going to ask the court for permission to keep you in the hospital, but at this point, you may choose to sign yourself in."

Because civil commitment entails a loss of freedom, the courts view the competing interests of citizen and state differently from those in other civil contests. In most civil lawsuits, each party is equal, and showing a preponderance of evidence usually is sufficient to win a case. In civil commitment, however, the state bears a higher burden of proof. According to the U.S. Supreme Court in *Addington v. Texas* (1979), the state must present "clear and convincing evidence" (a 75% probability of danger if the patient is not committed).

Commitment criteria

Each state defines its own commitment criteria, which usually include mental illness; danger to oneself, others, or property; inability to care for oneself; or grave disability and need of care. Medical and legal uses of such terms as *mentally ill* and *dangerous* may overlap. Consult the state statute for definitions and guidelines so that commitment forms will not be rejected on a technicality. Also, because commitment is a legal procedure, try to describe the patient in words that conform to the wording of the statute. "I think the patient might hurt someone" lacks the power of "This patient, suffering from schizophrenia characterized by homicidal command hallucinations, is a clear and present danger to others and is likely to be violent in the immediate future."

When commitment fails

A commitment application can be rejected, sometimes by a person with little clinical experience who has not examined the patient (such as a county mental health administrator). What implications does this have for your duties to the patient? Without a legal basis for detaining him, you must allow the patient to sign out of the emergency service; before he leaves, however, repeat the potential risks of forgoing treatment, and refer him to one or more psychiatric care settings that he may find acceptable. Finally, document all of your efforts in detail.

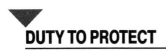

DUTY TO PROTECT

The basis for clinical services in emergency psychiatry is to protect the patient's health and welfare. In practice, a clinician commonly assists a patient in making decisions for the patient's own good, knowing that the psychiatric illness might cause the patient to harm himself or others. The patient's rights and the clinician's responsibilities might appear to be competing interests. Most of the time, however, they are compatible, with the patient volunteering for help and the clinician making recommendations that are acceptable to the patient. Problems arise when the clinician believes that the patient's mental illness may lead to suicide, homicide, injury, or destruction of property. In such cases, the clinician may need to exert the power of civil commitment to prevent a greater harm, at the expense of the patient's immediate liberty.

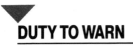

DUTY TO WARN

The duty to care for patients extends to the public in the sense that you have a duty to protect the public from dangerous acts carried out by your patients. This duty is based on case law from the 1970s and combines a public health principle (such as the duty to inform health authorities about a case of syphilis) with an aspect of law involving "special relationships." In the special relationship between clinician and patient, the clinician's duty to protect public safety supercedes that of confidentiality; thus, you may have a legal responsibility to warn the potential victim of a patient's violence. Be meticulous in documenting any actions you take, including consultations with colleagues, supervisors, administrators, or other authorities.

Tarasoff v. Regents of the University of California (1976) established the clinician's duty to warn a person who has been targeted as a victim by a homicidal patient. In this case, a university counseling service was judged to have failed in its duty to the victim, because the clinicians had sufficient knowledge of the patient's dangerousness to have detained him. Since *Tarasoff,* other cases have extended the duty to warn or protect to include unnamed or unknown victims and property (Simon, 1986), underscoring the importance of knowing the standards followed in your state. Understandably, from the clinician's point of view, the duty to warn or protect is complicated by the relative uncertainty of predicting dangerous behavior in mentally ill persons.

Because case law varies from state to state, you must become familiar with the standards of behavior expected of clinicians in your area. In California, for example, a clinician's liability for a patient's behavior is limited by statute, provided that all necessary steps were taken to protect the public. These steps can include hospitalizing the patient, reporting the situation to law enforcement authorities, or warning potential victims. Some states, however, approach a standard of "strict liability;" that is, the clinician is responsible for the patient's behavior even if he has taken all the necessary steps to protect the public.

LIABILITY

You can be held liable for harm caused by a patient to himself or others if you fail to recognize the need for intervention, leading to premature release; fail to take the necessary steps to protect a third party from a dangerous patient; provide inappropriate treatment (malpractice); or provide treatment without an informed consent (assault and battery). Any patient making a claim of malpractice must show evidence of negligence, harm, and causality, usually with the assistance of expert testimony. To prove negligence, the patient must show that you had a duty to care and that you breached the duty by providing services that fell below the standard of care required by the profession. To request damages (a monetary award), the patient must prove that harm was done, including the basic injury and subsequent related suffering. Finally, the patient must show causality, proving that the negligence directly caused the harm.

By practicing the fundamentals of sound clinical care, rather than intentionally defensive care, you usually will benefit the patient and minimize the potential for legal problems. The best strategy for avoiding a lawsuit after a bad outcome is to take responsibility (not blame) for your contribution, if any, explain what went wrong and why, and give the patient an opportunity to express his feelings. Being hostile, evasive, arrogant, or indifferent may cause the patient or family to file a lawsuit that they otherwise would not have filed. Involving a clinical supervisor, institutional administrator, or risk manager also can help resolve a clinical problem before it becomes a lawsuit.

Liability for postdischarge behavior

A psychiatric emergency service can be held accountable for the behavior of a patient it has discharged. This accountability lasts until another party or agency formally accepts responsibility for the patient, although the service can still be charged with negligent release if the patient subsequently harms himself or others and the service knew the patient was dangerous. Such liability can extend several months after discharge.

Consequently, discharge planning from a psychiatric emergency service must be conducted carefully. When a chain of custody is necessary between institutions, the referring agency is responsible for the patient until he arrives at the other institution. If questions of civil commitment arise, consult with legal authorities. If you suspect future dangerous behavior from a patient, emergency detention, followed by a formal hearing, is the safest action. If the patient is released, a clinician who says, "I didn't think he was committable," may not be protected from a claim of negligence.

Clinical approach

Although standards of conduct vary from state to state, consider the following recommendations to avoid any legal complications:
• Assess the patient for clinical signs of dangerousness, as described in Chapter 7, Violent Behavior.
• Document all findings, interventions, and reasons for any action taken. If you evaluate a patient for violent behavior and then discharge him, be sure to document your justification for the release.
• When in doubt, get help, first from a senior or supervising clinician, then from the appropriate legal authority. Because civil commitment is a legal process, don't hesitate to seek a ruling on

committability. If you are unsure about personal or institutional liability, contact the attorney for the emergency service or hospital.

• Remember that, if the court rejects civil commitment, you retain the duty to treat the patient and to warn any potential victims of the patient's violence.

• Continue to offer a reluctant patient opportunities to admit himself voluntarily.

• Maintain a tight chain of custody when referring a patient. A patient may agree to return for hospitalization ("I just need to go home for a few minutes to feed the cat") without intending to comply.

PATIENTS' RIGHTS

The concept of patients' rights is ingrained in the practice of institutional psychiatry. For patients in public institutions, these rights include treatment in the least restrictive environment, refusal of treatment, informed consent, freedom from abuse, and legal counsel. In the psychiatric emergency setting, you can apply these principles through your own policies and procedures, unless distinct local protocols, such as a Patient's Bill of Rights, are already in place. The patient's rights in the psychiatric emergency setting include:

• the right to leave the emergency service (unless the patient is dangerous or mentally incompetent)

• the right to refuse treatment (unless the patient is dangerous)

• the right to be informed about proposed treatments, their expected effects, and potential adverse effects

• the right to obtain legal counsel when a deprivation of liberty is at stake.

REFERENCES

Addington v. Texas. 441 US 418 (1979).

Simon, R.I. *Clinical Psychiatry and the Law.* Washington, D.C.: American Psychiatric Press, 1986.

Tarasoff v. Regents of the University of California. 17 Cal 3d 425, 131; Cal Rptr 14, 551 P 2d 334 (1976).

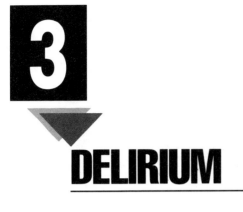

DELIRIUM

Undiagnosed medical illness in psychiatric patients is a major concern in clinical practice. Of patients who are referred for psychiatric treatment, 3.5% to 16% have an undetected medical illness (Dubin and Weiss, 1984). Of greater concern is the misdiagnosis of delirium as a psychiatric illness. Clinicians who focus predominantly on aberrant and often violent behavior might overlook medical illness as an underlying cause, with a resulting increase in patient morbidity and mortality. The mortality rate for delirium 3 months after diagnosis is 14 times greater than that for mood disorders (Weddington, 1982), and a hospitalized patient with delirium has a mortality rate 5.5 times greater than that of a patient diagnosed with dementia (Rabins and Folstein, 1982).

This chapter discusses the evaluation and differential diagnosis of acute organic mental disorder, emphasizing features of delirium that may superficially resemble functional psychiatric illness.

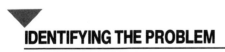

IDENTIFYING THE PROBLEM

Delirium is a reversible disturbance of cerebral metabolism secondary to a cerebral insult, such as an infection or metabolic disturbance. Onset is acute, usually within 4 to 6 hours, although it may evolve over several days or weeks. Delirium is characterized by impaired thinking, memory, perception, concentration, and attention (Lipowski, 1967).

In its most florid manifestation, delirium can be mistaken for a manic or schizophrenic episode. The agitated patient paces and cannot sit still. Thoughts are fragmented and incoherent. The patient expresses intense emotions, such as fear or anxiety, in response to delusions. For instance, he may refuse to leave a room or an area of the emergency department because "they'll know I'm here." Clinical evaluation is confounded further by fluctuating symptoms; within 30 minutes, the patient may be lethargic and no longer delusional. Thus, you must become familiar with the entire range of symptoms that occur in delirious patients.

Mental status findings

The *Diagnostic and Statistical Manual of Mental Disorders,* 3rd edition, revised *(DSM-III-R,* 1987) describes mental status findings common to patients with delirium.

Clouding of consciousness — the hallmark of delirium — can vary from loss of awareness of self and surroundings to stupor and coma. Most patients with delirium are lethargic or stuporous and tend to drowse or fall asleep while being interviewed. If this happens, try to arouse the patient by raising your voice or shaking him. In such situations, consider the patient delirious until proven otherwise.

You may be disconcerted by the patient's *fluctuating symptoms.* Lucid intervals, in which the patient is fully oriented and appears mentally intact, alternate with periods of significant cognitive impairment, in which the patient is suspicious, paranoid, and disoriented. Don't misinterpret fluctuating symptoms as willful attempts to deceive you.

Always consider *visual hallucinations* to be of organic etiology until all likely medical causes are ruled out. The hallucinations usually are colorful, vivid, and well defined. Visual hallucinations in younger patients should alert you to the possibility of drug or alcohol intoxication or withdrawal.

Illusions are misperceptions of an actual stimulus (for example, misinterpreting the sound of a dropped stethoscope for a gunshot or a crack in the wall for a snake). A significant correlation exists between illusions and an underlying medical illness.

The patient usually experiences *disorientation* to time and place but rarely, if ever, to person. The extent of the disorientation varies with the severity of the delirium.

A patient with delirium usually has *abnormal vital signs* (including tachycardia, sweating, fever, and dilated pupils) and *impaired attention span.* The patient is easily distracted by irrelevant stimuli and tends to shift from topic to topic in seemingly unrelated ways, his thoughts typically disjointed and incoherent. *Memory impairment* affects both short-term and long-term memory.

Sundowner's syndrome, a disturbance of the sleep-wake cycle, is characterized by drowsiness or stupor during the day and alertness and hypervigilance at night. The syndrome is most common in elderly patients with dementia (see Chapter 14, Geriatric Emergencies).

Rapidly changing *delusions* are another sign of delirium. The patient may initially say that "someone is out to get me" and then modify this to "someone is trying to poison my food" before affirming his belief that he is "dying of an incurable disease."

Agitation, another common sign, had been considered a requisite for a diagnosis of delirium. However, one can experience a "quiet" delirium, during which the patient appears calm and relaxed. Only through careful questioning can the clinician discover that the patient is disoriented, delusional, and hallucinatory.

Motor abnormalities (such as tremor, myoclonus, asterixis, and reflex and muscle tone changes) are exhibited by many, but not all, delirious patients (Wise, 1987). Other neurologic signs are relatively uncommon unless the delirium is caused by a primary central nervous system disturbance.

Physical findings

The initial physical examination of an agitated, delirious patient need not be intrusive or time-consuming. At a minimum, you should evaluate the patient's general appearance, vital signs, head (for injuries), eyes (for pupil size and for nystagmus or exophthalmos), neck (for rigidity or thyroid enlargement), skin color and perspiration, hands (for tremor, asterixis, or chorea), and reflexes (for hyperactivity or asymmetry). Ultimately, thorough medical and neurologic examinations are necessary to help determine the cause of the delirium (see *Delirium: Signs and causes,* page 26).

DELIRIUM: SIGNS AND CAUSES

SIGNS AND SYMPTOMS	POSSIBLE CAUSE
Elevated blood pressure	Hypertensive encephalopathy
Low blood pressure	Myocardial infarction
Tachycardia	Hypoglycemia, hypoxia, anemia, hyperthyroidism
Tachypnea	Chronic obstructive lung disease
Headache and stiff neck	Meningitis or intracranial hemorrhage
Nystagmus, ophthalmoplegia, and ataxia	Thiamine deficiency secondary to alcohol intake (Wernicke's encephalopathy)
Dilated pupils, tachycardia, flushing, and dry skin	Anticholinergic toxicity
Stupor or coma	Hypoglycemia (response to 50 ml of 50% dextrose and water I.V. will confirm diagnosis)
High fever, tachycardia, and hyperreflexia	Thyroid storm
Tachypnea, odor of acetone on breath, dehydration, and hypotension	Diabetic ketosis
Elevated autonomic signs, hyperreflexia, agitation, and visual hallucinations	Alcohol withdrawal syndrome
Fluctuating consciousness, history of head trauma, and dilated pupils (late sign)	Subdural hematoma
Ataxia, lethargy, and nystagmus	Phenytoin (Dilantin) toxicity
Memory disturbance, hallucinations, egocentricity, intense focusing of attention on some object, and automatisms	Complex partial seizures (temporal lobe epilepsy)

Source: Walker, 1983, p. 28. Adapted with permission from the publisher.

Laboratory studies

Order routine laboratory studies for any patient you suspect of having delirium to rule out life-threatening illnesses. These tests – complete blood count, glucose and electrolyte levels, blood urea nitrogen, chest X-ray, arterial blood gas levels, toxic drug screen, electrocardiogram, and serum drug levels (such as lithium and theophylline) – help detect problems that require immediate medical intervention.

A patient who exhibits acute behavioral changes or clouded consciousness that cannot be explained by laboratory evaluation may require a lumbar puncture. A computed tomography (CT) scan before the lumbar puncture helps rule out intracranial causes of delirium.

More extensive evaluation on an inpatient unit is necessary if the cause cannot be determined in the emergency setting. While the patient is hospitalized, additional laboratory testing may include a serial electroencephalogram; blood chemistries for heavy metals, thiamine, vitamin B_{12}, and folate levels; thyroid test; lupus erythematosus cell test; antinuclear antibody test; urine porphobilinogen; blood and urine cultures; and lumbar puncture and CT scan, if not performed earlier.

Differential diagnosis

The clinician may avoid searching for a cause because the etiologies of delirium are so diverse (Wise, 1987). Be especially alert to the most common life-threatening causes of delirium (see *Life-threatening causes of delirium,* page 28). Prescription medications are one of the most overlooked causes of delirium. Delirium in an elderly patient may be related to polypharmacy: The patient takes five or more medications a day, many of which are not needed. Simply discontinuing some of the medications or reducing the dosages may resolve the delirium.

At first glance, the symptoms of delirium may superficially resemble those of schizophrenia or mania. Too often the differential diagnosis is based on a single piece of data, a single symptom, a single item of past history, or a previous diagnosis (Leeman, 1975). An inexperienced clinician can easily be misled into a premature diagnosis of psychiatric illness (Dubin and Weiss, 1984). The pitfalls to diagnosis include:

LIFE-THREATENING CAUSES OF DELIRIUM

CAUSE	CLINICAL FINDINGS
Wernicke's encephalopathy or alcohol withdrawal syndrome	Ataxia, ophthalmoplegia, alcohol or drug history, elevated blood pressure or pulse rate, sweating, hyperreflexia
Hypertensive encephalopathy	Elevated blood pressure, papilledema
Hypoglycemia	History of insulin-dependent diabetes, decreased blood glucose
Hypoperfusion of the central nervous system	Decreased blood pressure, decreased cardiac output (for example, myocardial infarction, arrhythmia, cardiac failure), decreased hematocrit
Hypoxemia	History of pulmonary disease, decreased PO_2
Intracranial bleeding	History of unconsciousness or head trauma, focal neurologic signs
Meningitis or encephalitis	Meningeal signs, elevated white blood cell count, fever
Poisons or medications	Pupillary abnormality, nystagmus, ataxia

Source: Anderson, 1987, p. 425. Adapted with permission of the publisher.

- **Hallucinations and delusions.** These symptoms occur in many psychiatric syndromes, not only in delirium.
- **Agitation and violence.** These also are common symptoms. Violence commonly heralds an acute medical illness.
- **Patients who create their own diseases.** Alcoholics, drug users, and suicidal persons are patients for whom nonpsychiatrists have little tolerance. The pervasive feeling among many clinicians is that certain patients willfully bring illness upon themselves, diverting the clinician from "patients who really need my help."

■ **Psychiatric patients.** Nonpsychiatrists tend to minimize or ignore physical complaints in these patients. Even when patients have extensive psychiatric histories, reappearance of psychotic symptoms may indicate an organic disorder.

■ **Geriatric patients.** The complaints of elderly patients also tend to be minimized or disregarded by staff members, who assume that the problems result from senility or other conditions associated with old age.

▼ INTERPERSONAL INTERVENTION

Although interpersonal techniques alone cannot treat delirium, supportive therapy can help minimize a patient's agitation. Try to provide a quiet, reassuring atmosphere, and don't subject the patient to multiple interviews with medical students, interns, or residents. Keep your instructions direct and concise. To prevent an agitated or confused patient from harming himself or others, make sure that you, another staff member, or the patient's family or friends remain with him at all times.

Familiarity is a key to maintaining the patient's orientation. Reorient the patient periodically and tactfully, introducing yourself again and describing what you are doing and why (Tomb, 1988). A calm and sympathetic manner and the ability to anticipate the patient's anxiety by offering frequent reassurance helps reduce the patient's agitation (Tomb, 1988). Additionally, soft music from a radio or tape may help attenuate hypervigilance and agitation, particularly in a patient with sundowner's syndrome (Murray, 1987).

▼ PHARMACOLOGIC INTERVENTION

When a delirious patient becomes belligerent or assaultive, many clinicians erroneously withhold neuroleptic medication for fear that the drug will either obscure symptoms or place the patient in further medical jeopardy. As a result, mental status examinations, physical examinations, and diagnostic studies are sometimes performed on patients who are either mechanically restrained or held down by staff members. An examination performed in this manner is of questionable value, and the restraints themselves involve medical risks and complications. A patient with a cardiac illness or orthopedic problem, for example, may worsen his condition by struggling to free himself from the restraints. The argument that neuroleptic agents will obscure symptoms and delay diagnosis is specious because the definitive diagnosis is never made on a single mental status evaluation. Tranquilization of the patient is humane and clinically effective in ensuring behavioral control and reduces the risks of violence and self-injury.

Rapid tranquilization

Rapid tranquilization (RT) is a reliable procedure in which standard doses of a neuroleptic drug are administered at 30- to 60-minute intervals, with the dose titrated according to the patient's symptoms (Dubin et al., 1986). Target symptoms include excitement, anxiety, tension, hyperactivity, and agitation. At its best, RT can control hyperactivity and combativeness without restraints or isolation techniques. Core psychiatric symptoms, such as hallucinations and delusions, usually do not subside with short-term use of neuroleptics. RT is contraindicated in patients with an anticholinergic intoxication, as evidenced by dilated, unreactive pupils.

High-potency neuroleptic drugs are the preferred treatment; most patients usually respond to standard doses (see *Doses for rapid tranquilization*). Administer a test dose, noting the patient's behavioral response and any side effects. Avoid low-potency neuroleptic drugs, such as chlorpromazine (Thorazine) or thioridazine (Mellaril), because their strong anticholinergic side effects might exacerbate the delirium. Administer the medication in an oral concentrate form, if possible, rather than by intramuscular injection, which may agitate a patient or require the use of temporary restraints.

For delirious patients who do not respond to standard doses of neuroleptic agents during RT, Adams (1988) has proposed using a combination of haloperidol (Haldol) and lorazepam (Ativan). Side effects are usually few, mild, and reversible. The most common extrapyramidal symptoms are dystonia and akathisia.

DOSES FOR RAPID TRANQUILIZATION				
DRUG	**DOSE IN PATIENTS YOUNGER THAN 65**		**DOSE IN PATIENTS 65 OR OLDER**	
	Concentrate	I.M.	Concentrate	I.M.
thiothixene (Navane)	20 mg	10 mg	10 mg	5 mg
trifluoperazine (Stelazine)	20 mg	10 mg	10 mg	5 mg
haloperidol (Haldol)	10 mg	5 mg	5 mg	2.5 mg
loxapine (Loxitane)	25 mg	10 mg	15 mg	5 mg

Source: Dubin et al., 1986, p. 5. Adapted with permission of the publisher.

Intravenous RT

Intravenous RT, although not widely practiced by clinicians, may be of value in medical intensive care units when the patient's medical condition precludes the use of oral or intramuscular medication (Dubin et al., 1986). Several reports have documented the safety and efficacy of I.V. medication in medically ill and debilitated patients. I.V. administration may be useful in patients with lowered cardiac output who cannot absorb I.M. medication, those who are incapable of taking oral medication, and those with extensive tissue damage, such as burn patients.

I.V. antipsychotic medication can be safe and effective. Although onset of action varies, incidence of side effects from I.V. administration appears to be no greater than that from other routes. Some patients who receive I.V. neuroleptic drugs may actually have a lower incidence of extrapyramidal side effects than those receiving oral medication (Menza et al., 1987).

Treatment of neuroleptic side effects

Treatment for dystonia and akathisia is 2 mg of benztropine (Cogentin) or 50 mg of diphenhydramine (Benadryl) I.M. or I.V. Repeat the dose every 5 minutes for up to three doses. Relief usually occurs within 3 minutes of administration, although some patients, especially those with akathisia, may not respond. In these cases, 5 mg of diazepam (Valium) I.V. or 10 mg orally or 2 mg of lorazepam

I.V. or I.M. may be helpful. (See Chapter 6, Schizophrenia and Mania, for a more detailed discussion of RT and its side effects.)

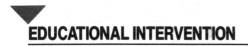

EDUCATIONAL INTERVENTION

Patient education cannot be attempted during a delirious episode, even in lucid intervals. And because a delirious patient will probably be transferred to an inpatient setting, you will not have much time to provide family members or friends with such information. When possible, briefly explain the problem (for instance, drug withdrawal, drug toxicity, suspected medical illness), and reassure them that the condition usually is short-lived. If the delirium was caused by drug use or dehydration, give them suggestions for preventing future episodes, such as closely monitoring all drugs purchased and periodically checking the house for medications or keeping a weekly weight chart and closely monitoring the patient's food and fluid intake.

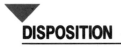

DISPOSITION

Most patients with delirium should be hospitalized. Their high risk of mortality necessitates comprehensive medical, neurologic, and psychiatric evaluations to ensure that all treatable causes are discovered. If you are certain that a patient's delirium results from an overuse of drugs or mild dehydration — and if a caring family member or friend is willing to stay with him overnight — you can discharge the patient and schedule him for a follow-up evaluation the next day. However, given the potentially grave prognosis for delirium, you may prefer to admit him to confirm the diagnosis and initiate appropriate treatment for the underlying cause.

MEDICOLEGAL CONSIDERATIONS

Failure to diagnose delirium will expose the patient to an excessive risk of morbidity and mortality. Although the common conception of delirium is a state of wildly disorganized behavior, it can be less dramatic. An elderly person with a delirium superimposed on dementia may exhibit only diminished verbal and motor behavior, as is commonly seen with infections. Cavalierly dismissing a confused patient as senile or demented rather than making an appropriate evaluation constitutes negligent care. Thus, for risk management purposes, document delirium as a possible diagnosis for any patient with disturbed consciousness.

Delirium is a medical emergency in which the patient is incompetent to participate in treatment decisions. With the family's knowledge and consent, you can begin treatment without a civil commitment decision. If a family member is unavailable and the delirium exposes the patient to an increased risk of morbidity or mortality, you can begin treatment without the family's consent.

REFERENCES

Adams, F. "Emergency Intravenous Sedation of the Delirious, Medically Ill Patient," *Journal of Clinical Psychiatry* 49(suppl):22-26, December 1988.

Anderson, W.H. "The Emergency Room," *Massachusetts General Hospital Handbook of General Hospital Psychiatry,* 2nd ed. Edited by Hackett, T.P., and Cassem, N.H. Littleton, Mass.: PSG Publishing Company, 1987.

Diagnostic and Statistical Manual of Mental Disorders, 3rd ed., revised. Washington, D.C.: American Psychiatric Association, 1987.

Dubin, W.R., and Weiss, K.J. "Diagnosis of Organic Brain Syndrome: An Emergency Department Dilemma," *Journal of Emergency Medicine* 1:393-397, 1984.

Dubin, W.R., et al. "Pharmacotherapy of Psychiatric Emergencies," *Journal of Clinical Psychopharmacology* 6(4):210-222, August 1986.

Dubin, W.R., et al. "Emergency Psychiatry," *Psychiatry* 2:5, 1986.

Leeman, C.P. "Diagnostic Errors in Emergency Room Medicine: Physical Illness in Patients Labeled 'Psychiatric' and Vice Versa," *International Journal of Psychiatry in Medicine* 6(4):533-540, 1975.

Lipowski, Z.J. "Delirium, Clouding of Consciousness, and Confusion," *Journal of Nervous and Mental Disease* 145:227-255, 1967.

Menza, M.A., et al. "Decreased Extrapyramidal Symptoms with Intravenous Haloperidol," *Journal of Clinical Psychiatry* 48(7):278-280, July 1987.

Murray, G.B. "Confusion, Delirium, and Dementia," in *Massachusetts General Hospital Handbook of General Hospital Psychiatry,* 2nd ed. Edited by Hackett, T.P., and Cassem, N.H. Littleton, Mass.: PSG Publishing Company, 1987.

Rabins, P.V., and Folstein, M.F. "Delirium and Dementia: Diagnostic Criteria and Fatality Rates," *British Journal of Psychiatry* 140:149-153, February 1982.

Tomb, D.A. *Psychiatry for the House Officer.* Baltimore: Williams and Wilkins, 1988.

Walker, J.I. *Psychiatric Emergencies: Intervention and Resolution.* Philadelphia: J.B. Lippincott, 1983.

Weddington, W.W. "The Mortality of Delirium: An Underappreciated Problem?" *Psychosomatics* 23(12):1232-1235, December 1982.

Wise, M.G. "Delirium," in *Textbook of Neuropsychiatry.* Edited by Hales, R.E., and Yudofsky, S.C. Washington: American Psychiatric Press, 1987.

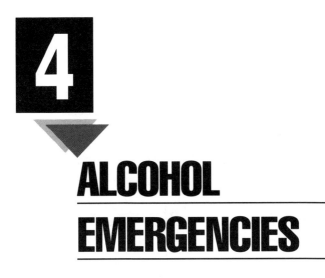

ALCOHOL
EMERGENCIES

Alcohol-related crises are among the most prevalent psychiatric emergencies, accounting for 20% to 36% of visits to emergency departments (Walker, 1983) and nearly 40% of admissions to general medical and surgical wards (Hanke, 1984). Aside from the medical complications of alcoholism, these emergencies include alcohol intoxication, idiosyncratic intoxication, alcohol withdrawal, alcohol amnestic disorder, and alcohol hallucinosis.

IDENTIFYING THE PROBLEM: ALCOHOL INTOXICATION

An intoxicated patient exhibits a range of behaviors and physical symptoms, depending on the amount of alcohol in the blood.

Mental status findings
Mild to moderate symptoms include loquacity, slurred speech, impaired judgment, shortened attention span, inappropriate emotional responses, and euphoria (Gallant, 1989). A more severely intoxicated patient may become irrational, angry, or violent; display pro-

gressively sluggish responses to environmental stimuli; and have the "dry heaves."

Physical findings

Physical findings in a patient with mild to moderate intoxication include alcohol on the breath, diminished motor coordination, dysmetria, ataxia, nystagmus, blurred vision, dizziness, flushed face, orthostatic hypotension, hematemesis, and stupor. In cases of severe intoxication, the patient has a decreased respiratory rate, slow pulse, low blood pressure, sluggish reflexes, and low body temperature; in the most serious cases, a patient can progress to shock and coma.

Laboratory studies

Depending on the patient's medical history and on clinical findings at the time of evaluation, laboratory studies may include a complete blood count (for hematemesis), an electrocardiogram (ECG) and electrolyte studies (for cardiac abnormalities), a hepatic profile (for jaundice), and a serum glucose level and computed tomography (CT) scan (for persistent stupor).

Differential diagnosis

Alcohol intoxication can resemble many serious medical diseases, including diabetic ketoacidosis, hypoglycemia, intoxication with barbiturates or other sedative and hypnotic agents, subdural hematoma, multiple sclerosis, cerebellar ataxia, and Huntington's chorea (Dubin and Stolberg, 1981). If the patient is uncooperative and hostile, you can easily overlook potential medical complications of alcohol abuse, including cardiac arrhythmia, cardiac failure, upper and lower GI tract bleeding, pneumonia, liver failure or associated ascites, pancreatitis, anemia, subdural hematoma, seizures, and peripheral neuropathy (Schuckit, 1989). To elicit alcohol-related medical problems, Walker (1983) suggests asking the following questions:
• Did the patient have convulsions?
• Did the patient drink alcohol in combination with medications or drugs?
• Does the patient have a history of alcohol withdrawal syndrome, ulcer disease, heart disease, or diabetes?
• Was the patient recently involved in an accident?
• Did the patient suffer a recent head injury?

- Does the patient have evidence of GI bleeding?

Head injury is of special concern because intoxicated patients may be unable to feel the site of pain. Carefully examine the patient for bruises, cuts, and fractures, and closely examine the patient's scalp for evidence of traumatic head injury.

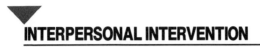

INTERPERSONAL INTERVENTION

Perhaps no patient draws more negative response from hospital staff members than an intoxicated patient. Although such reactions are a normal response to the annoying behavior and mayhem created by an intoxicated person, you cannot allow these personal feelings to influence your professional judgments and actions.

Before interviewing a loud and boisterous patient, alert the hospital security force. Although security intervention is seldom required, you may find it reassuring to have the assistance ready. Conduct the interview in a large, comfortable room. Many alcoholic patients are claustrophobic, and you may be uncomfortable in an enclosed room with a potentially violent patient.

Assume a tolerant, nonthreatening manner. An authoritarian position is much more likely to precipitate a violent outburst (see Chapter 7, Violent Behavior). Also be prepared to tolerate insults and threats and not personalize them.

Approach the patient with an introductory handshake, and make no efforts to change the patient's behavior (Hackett, 1987). Listening to a patient's tirade and attempting to make sense of it is more effective than demanding that he speak more temperately, especially for uncovering a major grievance or misunderstanding. Try to avoid direct eye contact for more than a few seconds, because an intoxicated patient commonly interprets this as a challenge. Offering food, coffee, or juice may be helpful (Hackett, 1987); many patients are less aggressive after eating.

PHARMACOLOGIC INTERVENTION

If the patient is excited or potentially assaultive, a benzodiazepine, such as diazepam (Valium) 5 mg orally every 30 to 60 minutes, is recommended (Hackett, 1987). If the patient is so agitated that he refuses to take oral medication, 1 to 2 mg of lorazepam (Ativan) may be given intramuscularly every hour until the patient is calm. Dosage requirements vary and commonly must be determined empirically. If the patient has a concomitant psychotic illness, a high-potency neuroleptic agent can be administered as an oral concentrate or intramuscularly every 30 to 60 minutes for up to six doses a day. Recommended doses are thiothixene (Navane), 10 mg I.M. or 20 mg concentrate; haloperidol (Haldol), 5 mg I.M. or 10 mg concentrate; and loxapine (Loxitane), 10 mg I.M. or 25 mg concentrate.

▼

EDUCATIONAL INTERVENTION

One of the cornerstones of treatment for alcohol addiction is educating the patient about the disease and its diverse effects on him and on his family and associates. Unfortunately, several factors inhibit educational efforts in the emergency setting: an intoxicated person is not receptive to learning, and an alcoholic who continues to drink usually denies his illness vehemently.

Because discharging an intoxicated patient is clinically and legally risky, the safe course is to give him time to "sleep it off" and then attempt educational interventions. If possible, have a representative of Alcoholics Anonymous speak with the patient to reduce his denial. When speaking with the patient yourself, cover the following points:

• Alcoholism is a disease.

• Abstinence is the only way to recover.

• Most people need support (such as from Alcoholics Anonymous) to achieve and maintain abstinence.

• The effects of alcoholism are already apparent (the current emergency).

• Continued drinking is certain to destroy the quality of the patient's life and may cause premature death.

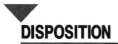

DISPOSITION

Because alcohol intoxication is a time-limited condition, most patients can be discharged to outpatient care. When possible, send the patient home in the company of family members or friends, with referral to an alcohol treatment program the next day. If the patient is already an active member of Alcoholics Anonymous (AA), obtain his permission to call the AA sponsor to arrange for immediate reinvolvement in AA.

No patient who remains ataxic should be discharged from the emergency setting, and hospitalization is recommended for intoxicated patients who have concomitant medical disorders, such as diabetes, dehydration, hypertension, or head injury, or who are suffering from medical complications of alcoholism.

IDENTIFYING THE PROBLEM: IDIOSYNCRATIC INTOXICATION

The essential feature of idiosyncratic intoxication is altered behavior, usually aggression, caused by ingesting an amount of alcohol that would be insufficient to induce intoxication in most people. Anterograde amnesia (an inability to learn new information) usually occurs for the duration of the intoxication (*DSM-III-R*, 1987). The patient's behavior during intoxication is atypical of his behavior when sober. Behavioral changes may last several hours or days and usually end in a prolonged sleep (Hackett, 1987).

Mental status findings
Mental status findings in a patient who is idiosyncratically intoxicated include agitation, impulsiveness, and aggression. At times, the patient may be delusional or experience visual hallucinations. Hyperactivity, restlessness, and anxiousness are also common.

Physical findings
No characteristic physical findings are helpful in diagnosing idiosyncratic intoxication.

Laboratory studies

Useful tests for making the diagnosis are an electroencephalogram, drug screen, and CT head scan.

Differential diagnosis

The differential diagnosis should exclude temporal lobe epilepsy, intoxication from other drugs, drug withdrawal, and malingering.

INTERPERSONAL INTERVENTION

Because you cannot predict whether the patient will become aggressive, consider the patient dangerous and use caution during the initial examination. Gallant (1989) suggests the following guidelines for managing patients with idiosyncratic intoxication:

• Never disagree with the patient. An individual on the verge of explosive behavior can be set off by any discord.

• Speak calmly and slowly with no sudden change in voice tone or pitch.

• Initiate physical movement slowly, and keep it to a minimum.

• Learn the patient's first name and use it, which may make the patient feel more comfortable.

• Remember that the longer your dialogue with the patient continues, the less likely he is to become violent. Toward this end, try to discover personal details about the patient. If he mentions certain people who seem to elicit positive feelings, ask him for permission to contact these people and bring them into the dialogue.

PHARMACOLOGIC INTERVENTION

If the patient requires sedation, 10 mg of diazepam I.V. over 1 to 2 minutes or 1 to 2 mg of lorazepam I.V. over 1 to 2 minutes is recommended (Gallant, 1989). These doses can be repeated at 10-minute intervals. An alternative would be 5 mg of haloperidol I.M., repeated every hour if necessary (Schuckit, 1989).

EDUCATIONAL INTERVENTION

Because amnesia usually accompanies idiosyncratic intoxication, reserve educational interventions until the patient is lucid and attentive. At that time, describe the patient's behavior to him in detail. Although your description may induce in him a sense of shame, the negative feeling may help him remain abstinent. Other messages about the disease of alcoholism may or may not be relevant, depending on his history. The typical patient with this disorder does not ingest much alcohol, but its dangers are nevertheless potent. Make this clear to the patient by saying, "Alcohol poisons your brain. You seem to be one of those people who cannot drink, even in small amounts. If you do, you are playing with fire."

DISPOSITION

Usually, the patient can be discharged once the episode is over. If the patient remains agitated or delusional, however, admit him for further psychiatric evaluation. Refer a patient who cannot control his drinking to an alcohol rehabilitation program.

IDENTIFYING THE PROBLEM: ALCOHOL WITHDRAWAL

Heavy drinkers experience various withdrawal symptoms when they stop drinking or drastically reduce alcohol intake. Withdrawal symptoms can be precipitated by severe physical stress, such as pneumonia, or the need for a major medical or surgical procedure for which the patient must be hospitalized, leading to a forced withdrawal.

Mental status findings

Symptoms of uncomplicated alcohol withdrawal peak 24 to 48 hours after the last drink and subside within 5 to 7 days, even without treatment. However, mild irritability and insomnia may last for 10 days or more. Patients in withdrawal usually are depressed, irritable, and anxious and may experience transient hallucinations or illusions.

The mental status of a patient with alcohol withdrawal syndrome (a severe form of withdrawal formerly known as delirium tremens) is similar to that of a delirious patient. A patient typically experiences vivid visual hallucinations. Tactile, olfactory, and auditory hallucinations also can occur. Hallucinations usually are frightening—the patient sees and feels mice or lice crawling on the skin, or he sees animals, especially snakes, in threatening poses (Hackett, 1987). Other signs of alcohol withdrawal syndrome include disorientation to time, place, or person; waxing and waning of symptoms; and intermittent agitation, commonly violent in nature.

Physical findings

Physical findings—the prominent feature of alcohol withdrawal and the most helpful in establishing the diagnosis—include tachycardia, sweating, elevated blood pressure, nausea, vomiting, malaise, weakness, tremulousness, hyperreflexia, orthostatic hypotension, and, occasionally, generalized seizures.

Left untreated, alcohol withdrawal syndrome can lead to death secondary to infections, fat emboli, or cardiac arrhythmias associated with hyperkalemia, hyperpyrexia, poor hydration, and hypertension (Frances and Franklin, 1987). The syndrome usually occurs in those with a 5- to 15-year history of heavy drinking who decrease their blood alcohol levels and who have a significant physical illness, such as infection, trauma, liver disease, or metabolic disorder (Frances and Franklin, 1987). Onset ranges from 24 to 72 hours after cessation of drinking.

Laboratory studies

The initial laboratory evaluation consists of blood glucose levels, serum drug levels, complete blood count (CBC), urinalysis, and serum electrolytes. Other laboratory studies that may be helpful are an ECG, chest X-ray, serum amylase, arterial blood gas (ABG) studies, and CT scan (if head trauma is suspected or found).

Differential diagnosis

Differential diagnosis for alcohol withdrawal and for the more severe alcohol withdrawal syndrome must rule out concomitant medical illness (see *Common nonalcoholic causes of delirium,* page 44). After these medical illnesses are excluded, the primary differential diagnoses are essential tremor, withdrawal from sedative or hypnotic agents, hypoglycemia, and diabetic ketoacidosis (*DSM-III-R,* 1987). Hackett (1987) cautions that a clinician can easily overlook alcohol withdrawal as a diagnosis when the patient's manner, social position, or reputation belie the possibility of alcoholism.

▼
INTERPERSONAL INTERVENTION

Most patients undergoing mild alcohol withdrawal respond well to reassurance and acceptance. Staff members must treat these patients with tolerance and try to suppress any negative feelings they may have for patients with alcohol disorders. Additionally, relatives and friends can be a useful adjunct to treatment because they provide support and familiarity to the patient. Mild, pleasurable sensory stimulation, such as soft music, may further reduce the patient's agitation (Gallant, 1989).

Be clear and unambiguous with the patient at all times, identifying yourself as often as necessary and explaining the procedures that must be carried out (Tomb, 1988). Keep the patient in a well-lighted room, under constant observation by staff, family members, or friends to prevent him from wandering or sustaining injury.

Unfortunately, interpersonal interventions have limited value for a patient with alcohol withdrawal syndrome, but you should try to be tolerant and supportive, minimize stimulation, identify yourself periodically, explain any procedures you must perform, and be clear, direct, and concise in your instructions.

▼
PHARMACOLOGIC INTERVENTION

The drug of choice for treating patients in alcohol withdrawal is a benzodiazepine (Schuckit, 1989). Other drugs—including clonidine (Catapres), propranolol (Inderal), atenolol (Tenormin), haloperidol, chlorpromazine (Thorazine), and hydroxyzine (Atarax)—have been used but are not recommended for routine therapy of alcohol withdrawal.

COMMON NONALCOHOLIC CAUSES OF DELIRIUM

Medical
(infection, thyrotoxicosis, hypoparathyroidism, congestive heart failure)

Surgical
(head trauma, postanesthesia confusional state, brain tumor, fat embolus, pancreatitis)

Metabolic
(hypoxia, uremia, hypoglycemia, hepatic encephalopathy, water intoxication)

Drug ingestion
(bromides, steroids, stimulants, atropine, psychedelics)

Drug withdrawal
(barbiturates, tranquilizers, opiates)

Source: Usdin and Lewis, 1979, p. 329. Reprinted with permission of the publisher.

The primary decision in administering benzodiazepines is whether to use long- or short-acting medication. Long-acting medications, such as diazepam or chlordiazepoxide (Librium), ease withdrawal because of their long half-lives but can result in drug accumulation, which can cause lethargy, drowsiness, and ataxia, especially in a patient with hepatic impairment. Short-acting benzodiazepines, which are less likely to accumulate, must be administered more frequently because their short half-life results in rapid disappearance from the plasma, which can worsen alcohol withdrawal syndrome and precipitate seizures.

Additionally, patients in alcohol withdrawal should receive vitamin and mineral supplements, because vitamin deficiencies are common in those with chronic alcoholism (Frances and Franklin, 1987). A suggested regimen consists of thiamine (100 mg P.O. four times daily), folic acid (1 mg P.O. four times daily), a daily multivitamin, and magnesium sulfate (1 g I.M. every 6 hours for 2 days if status postwithdrawal seizures occur).

Alcohol withdrawal seizures

From 1% to 4% of patients in alcohol withdrawal experience seizures (Schuckit, 1989). These seizures, associated with long-term

DRUG TREATMENT OF ALCOHOL WITHDRAWAL SEIZURES

DRUG	INTERVENTION
diazepam (Valium)	Administer 10 mg I.V. over 1 to 2 minutes; repeat until the seizure clears. Do not exceed 30 mg of diazepam over 15 to 20 minutes.
amobarbital (Amytal)	Administer 100 to 150 mg/minute I.V. unless respiration is compromised. Repeat until the seizure clears.
phenytoin (Dilantin)	Administer 1,000 mg I.V. over 20 minutes (50 ml/minute in a glucose-free normal saline solution).

Source: Gallant, 1989; Frances and Franklin, 1988.

drinking, appear 7 to 38 hours after the last drink, with the average onset at 24 hours. More than 50% of patients with alcohol withdrawal seizures endure bursts of two to six generalized seizures, although less than 3% of these patients progress to status epilepticus (Frances and Franklin, 1987). Because alcohol withdrawal seizures do not represent a primary seizure disorder, a patient without such a disorder should not be routinely placed on anticonvulsant medication. Phenytoin (Dilantin) does not give added protection against seizures beyond that provided by the benzodiazepines. (See *Drug treatment of alcohol withdrawal seizures.*)

Alcohol withdrawal syndrome

The primary pharmacologic intervention is sedation to attenuate the severity of the withdrawal. A regimen of benzodiazepines – including chlordiazepoxide, diazepam, oxazepam (Serax), and lorazepam – is usually advised. Neuroleptic medications should be used only for the most severe symptoms, such as agitation or hallucinations that do not respond to benzodiazepines. Neuroleptic agents do not increase incidence of seizures (Benforado and Houden, 1979; Lenchan et al., 1985). Neuroleptic doses are similar to those used in rapid tranquilization: haloperidol, 5 mg I.M. or 10

MANAGING ALCOHOL WITHDRAWAL SYNDROME

PROCEDURE	CONSIDERATIONS
Administer vitamins.	Thiamine, 100 mg I.M. followed by 100 mg P.O. for 3 consecutive days; folic acid, 1 mg/day; multiple-vitamin tablets, 1 /day.
Sedate the patient.	Benzodiazepines are recommended.
Administer fluids as needed.	Carefully individualize and titrate (overhydration is common).
Administer potassium chloride.	If serum potassium is low and the patient has normal kidney function, replace with potassium chloride.
Administer 50% magnesium sulfate, 2 to 4 ml I.M. every 8 hours for three doses.	Magnesium deficiency can contribute to lethargy and weakness and lower the patient's seizure threshold.
Consider anticonvulsants.	Anticonvulsants are necessary only if the patient has a history of seizures or is in status epilepticus.
Provide a high-carbohydrate diet.	Hypoglycemia is a significant danger in abstinent alcoholic patients.

Source: Walker, 1983. Adapted with permission of the publisher.

mg concentrate; thiothixene, 10 mg I.M. or 20 mg concentrate; loxapine, 10 mg I.M. or 25 mg concentrate; or fluphenazine (Prolixin), 5 mg I.M. or 10 mg concentrate.

Adjunct therapy consists of vitamins and minerals. Thiamine is necessary to prevent development of alcohol amnestic disorder. Potassium supplements are prescribed for fatigue and muscle weakness, and magnesium is given to raise the seizure threshold. No evidence suggests that anticonvulsants will protect a patient from withdrawal seizures; therefore, they should be prescribed only if the patient has an underlying seizure disorder. (See *Managing alcohol withdrawal syndrome.*)

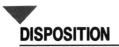

EDUCATIONAL INTERVENTION

Educational interventions for alcohol withdrawal are similar to those for alcohol intoxication (see page 38).

DISPOSITION

Outpatient medical detoxification is possible for most patients undergoing mild withdrawal, although close follow-up care, including daily visits, is essential to ensure adequate hydration and prevent complications. Outpatient treatment permits the patient to remain in work and social settings, and family members can provide much-needed support. If possible, the patient should be discharged in the company of friends or relatives.

Hospitalization may be necessary if the patient has:
• hallucinosis
• seizures
• temperature greater than 101° F (38.3° C)
• head trauma leading to unconsciousness
• clouded sensorium
• serious medical illness
• history of delirium, psychosis, or seizures in previous untreated withdrawals.

Note: Because alcohol withdrawal syndrome is life-threatening, a patient with this condition should be admitted to the hospital for aggressive medical intervention.

IDENTIFYING THE PROBLEM: ALCOHOL AMNESTIC DISORDER

Alcohol amnestic disorder is associated with excessive alcohol consumption and a diet deficient in vitamins, especially thiamine. Although most often associated with alcoholism, this disorder can occur with malabsorption syndrome, severe anorexia, upper GI tract obstruction, prolonged intravenous feeding, thyrotoxicosis, and hemodialysis (Frances and Franklin, 1987).

Historically, alcohol amnestic disorder has been referred to as Wernicke-Korsakoff syndrome, which is actually two separate disorders: Wernicke's encephalopathy (characterized by neurologic dysfunction) and Korsakoff's psychosis (characterized by severe memory impairment). Korsakoff's psychosis, the amnestic disorder, usually follows an acute episode of Wernicke's encephalopathy.

Mental status findings

Mental status findings characteristic of Korsakoff's psychosis are retrograde amnesia (an inability to remember events that occurred several years before onset of the illness) and anterograde amnesia (an inability to learn new information). In its acute stage, the deficiency is striking—patients cannot recall the day, time, or the examiner's first name, even after being given this information several times (Hackett, 1987). Patients usually are cheerful, pleasant, and unaware of the memory loss. Those with Wernicke's encephalopathy are disoriented and either apathetic or profoundly lethargic, at times progressing to coma.

Physical findings

Physical findings include cerebellar ataxia with a broad-based gait (the patient's legs are much wider apart when walking to maintain balance), inability to perform the finger-to-nose test, and oculomotor disturbances, which may include deficiency in conjugate gaze, horizontal and vertical nystagmus, and ptosis.

Laboratory studies

Standard tests include those for patients with organic disorders: a CBC, electrolyte studies, ECG, glucose, BUN level, and chest X-ray. Additionally, thiamine, folate, and vitamin B_{12} levels should be determined.

Differential diagnosis

The chief differential diagnosis is between delirium and dementia. Patients with alcohol amnestic disorder do not experience a clouding of consciousness as do those with delirium and intoxication. Despite the memory loss, general intellectual ability remains intact, in contrast to alcohol dementia or Alzheimer's disease (Gallant, 1989).

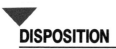

INTERPERSONAL INTERVENTION

The primary interpersonal intervention is careful observation to prevent the patient from wandering or harming himself. Additionally, staff members should be supportive, reassuring, and tolerant.

PHARMACOLOGIC INTERVENTION

Wernicke's encephalopathy is a medical emergency. Failure to treat the coma resulting from this disorder can increase risk of mortality. Further, the longer the coma remains untreated, the poorer the prognosis. Thus, the patient should receive 100 mg of thiamine I.M. daily for at least 3 days, followed by oral multivitamin preparations (Schuckit, 1989). The patient's oculomotor signs usually improve several hours after receiving thiamine. If not, they may be a result of hypomagnesemia (Frances and Franklin, 1987). In such instances, 1 to 2 ml of magnesium sulfate I.M. in a 50% solution should be administered. When any intoxicated patient is given I.V. glucose, thiamine should either be given I.M. or added to the I.V. solution to prevent the development of the amnestic disorder. The patient should also receive a balanced diet and 100 mg of oral thiamine three times daily.

EDUCATIONAL INTERVENTION

Educational inteventions for alcohol amnestic disorder are similar to those for alcohol intoxication (see page 38).

DISPOSITION

In view of the potentially serious prognosis, a patient with alcohol amnestic disorder should be admitted to the hospital. In an inpatient setting, the patient can safely be withdrawn from alcohol and given aggressive treatment for vitamin and mineral deficiencies.

▼

IDENTIFYING THE PROBLEM: ALCOHOL HALLUCINOSIS

Alcohol hallucinosis is characterized by vivid and persistent hallucinations that develop in alcohol-dependent persons within 48 hours after they stop drinking or reduce their alcohol intake, although hallucinations can occur in patients who continue to drink (Hackett, 1987). The disorder, which can last for several weeks or months, primarily affects those who have been heavy drinkers for 10 or more years (*DSM-III-R,* 1987).

Mental status findings

Mental status findings include vivid auditory and visual hallucinations, the key features of alcohol hallucinosis. Auditory hallucinations are more common, typically in the form of voices discussing the patient. The voices may threaten or malign the patient, accusing men of homosexual practices or women of promiscuity, and the patient may respond to auditory commands. At times, a frightening delusion can develop in response to hallucinations, leading patients to call the police or arm themselves. In extreme cases, patients may commit suicide (Hackett, 1987). Chronic alcohol hallucinosis is identified by ideas of reference, poorly systematized persecutory delusions, tangential thinking, and inappropriate affect.

Physical findings

No physical findings specific to alcohol hallucinosis exist, although findings characteristic of alcohol abuse may be evident on examination.

Laboratory studies

No specific laboratory studies facilitate the diagnosis.

Differential diagnosis

Alcohol hallucinosis can be differentiated from paranoid schizophrenia on the basis of heavy alcohol use, lack of formal thought disorder (unless it has progressed to a chronic stage), and lack of schizophrenia or mania as a part of the family history (Frances and Franklin, 1987). Hallucinations typical of this disorder, unlike those of alcohol withdrawal, occur despite intact orientation and memory and lack of autonomic arousal (Frances and Franklin, 1987).

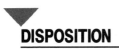

INTERPERSONAL INTERVENTION

Patience and kindness are fundamental interpersonal interventions. Try to remain supportive and nonjudgmental when caring for these patients.

PHARMACOLOGIC INTERVENTION

Although signs and symptoms resolve spontaneously within several weeks, neuroleptic drugs are useful for reducing agitation and promoting patient comfort until the psychosis clears (Schuckit, 1988). Recommended doses of oral neuroleptic agents include haloperidol, 2 to 5 mg; thiothixene, 5 to 10 mg; loxapine, 10 to 25 mg; or fluphenazine, 2 to 5 mg. All doses are given twice daily. Neuroleptic agents should not be given for more than 4 weeks; periodically reassess the patient so that medications can be discontinued when psychotic thinking abates.

EDUCATIONAL INTERVENTION

Educational interventions for alcohol hallucinosis are similar to those for alcohol intoxication (see page 38).

DISPOSITION

A patient with alcohol hallucinosis should be admitted to the hospital and withdrawn from alcohol. Because of the frightening nature of the hallucinations, admit the patient for observation for 24 to 48 hours to prevent possible harm to the patient or others.

▼

MEDICOLEGAL CONSIDERATIONS

Alcoholic emergencies commonly involve two legal issues: competence and dangerousness. Usually, patients with idiosyncratic intoxication, alcohol withdrawal syndrome, amnestic disorders, or hallucinosis are not competent. Many such patients are uncooperative, combative, psychotic, or lacking insight, which further complicates treatment. You have a duty to ensure appropriate care for intoxicated patients and can initiate treatment without consent for patients in critical situations, such as those experiencing delirium or hallucinosis. When possible, ask family members to give their consent for treatment, additional patient history, and direct support to the patient.

Intoxicated persons are at great risk for harming themselves, others, or property, according to reports from the Drug Abuse Warning Network, which correlates alcohol and drug use with hospital emergency visits and deaths reported to county medical examiners (National Institute on Drug Abuse, 1987). Make every effort to detain an intoxicated patient until he is sober and to discharge the patient in the care of relatives, friends, or AA members. You can be held legally responsible for harm caused by an intoxicated patient you release too soon.

REFERENCES

Benforado, J.M., and Houden, D. "The Use of Haloperidol to Control Agitation/ Violence during Admission to an Alcohol Detoxification Center," *Currents in Alcoholism* 7:331-338, 1979.

Diagnostic and Statistical Manual of Mental Disorders, 3rd ed., revised. Washington, D.C.: American Psychiatric Association, 1987.

Dubin, W.R., and Stolberg, R. *Emergency Psychiatry for the House Officer.* Bridgeport, Conn.: Robert B. Luce Inc., 1981.

Frances, R.J., and Franklin, J.E. "Alcohol-induced Organic Mental Disorders," in *Textbook of Neuropsychiatry.* Edited by Hales, R.E., and Yudofsky, S.C. Washington, D.C.: American Psychiatric Press, Inc., 1987.

Gallant, D.M. "Treatment of Organic Mental Disorders," in *Treatments of Psychiatric Disorders: A Task Force Report of the American Psychiatric Association.* Washington, D.C.: American Psychiatric Association, 1989.

Hackett, T.P. "Alcoholism: Acute and Chronic States," in *Massachusetts General Hospital Handbook of General Hospital Psychiatry,* 2nd ed. Edited by Hackett, T.P., and Cassem, N.H. Littleton, Mass.: PSG Publishing Company, Inc., 1987.

Hanke, N. *Handbook of Emergency Psychiatry.* Lexington, Mass.: The Collamore Press, 1984.

Lenchan, G.P., et al. "Use of Haloperidol in the Management of Agitated or Violent Alcohol-Intoxicated Patients in the Emergency Department: A Pilot Study," *Journal of Emergency Nursing* 11:72-79, 1985.

National Institute on Drug Abuse. "Trends in Drug Abuse-Related Hospital Emergency Room Episodes and Medical Examiner Cases for Selected Drugs: Drug Abuse Warning Network (DAWN) 1976 to 1985, Series H, #3. Rockville, Md.: United States Department of Health and Human Services, 1987.

Schuckit, M.A. *Drug and Alcohol Abuse: A Clinical Guide to Diagnosis and Treatment,* 3rd ed. New York: Plenum Medical Book Company, 1989.

Tomb, D.A. *Psychiatry for the House Officer,* 3rd ed. Baltimore: Williams and Wilkins, 1988.

Usdin, G., and Lewis, J.M., eds. *Psychiatry in General Medical Practice.* New York: McGraw-Hill Book Company, 1979.

Walker, J.I. *Psychiatric Emergencies: Intervention and Resolution.* Philadelphia: J.B. Lippincott, 1983.

5

DRUG
ABUSE
EMERGENCIES

Diagnosing drug abuse emergencies can be difficult, especially when the patient is psychotic from intoxication or delirious from withdrawal. Precise diagnosis can also be hindered if the patient has abused several substances or has an underlying psychiatric illness. Concurrent medical illness or injury can complicate the clinical picture by augmenting the drug's effect or masking the usual symptoms. In addition, a patient in withdrawal may have been ingesting drugs, thus obscuring signs and symptoms.

The drug of abuse cannot be established without a laboratory analysis of a drug sample and, when possible, the patient's body fluids and stomach contents. Even if the patient can identify the drug taken, a laboratory analysis is necessary to confirm the drug's identity, determine its dosage and purity, and detect contaminants. Despite its inherent difficulties, a diagnostic approach that includes mental status, physical, and neurologic findings can help establish the drug of abuse (see *Triage approach to drug abuse,* pages 56 and 57). This chapter reviews intoxication and withdrawal syndromes of the major classes of abused drugs.

▼
IDENTIFYING THE PROBLEM: STIMULANT ABUSE

Stimulant abuse, which has reached epidemic proportions in the United States, can lead to intoxication, delirium, or an organic delusional syndrome. Commonly abused stimulants include amphetamine, benzphetamine (Didrex), caffeine (No-Doz), cocaine, dextroamphetamine (Dexedrine), methamphetamine (Desoxyn), methylphenidate (Ritalin), phenmetrazine (Preludin), and phentermine (Ionamin).

Mental status findings

Symptoms of acute stimulant abuse include a heightened sense of well-being, increased sense of alertness, decreased anxiety, reduced social inhibitions, increased talkativeness, and poor judgment manifested by loss of money, sexual indiscretion, and illegal activities (Gawin and Ellinwood, 1989). The patient's symptoms usually resolve within 48 hours. When stimulant intoxication progresses to delirium, the patient exhibits grandiosity, psychomotor agitation, paranoid ideation, formication (sensation of insects crawling on the skin), bizarre behavior (such as sorting objects into various groups), stereotypical movements of the mouth and tongue (such as teeth grinding, lip biting, and skin picking), tactile or visual hallucinations, and distorted perceptions, including command hallucinations to harm oneself or others (*DSM-III-R*, 1987). Delusional states can also develop. In such cases, patients have temporary but dramatic paranoid delusions while remaining alert and fully oriented.

Physical findings

Physical findings include tachycardia, hypertension, hyperthermia, dilated pupils, perspiration or chills, hyperreflexia, nausea, and vomiting. You must conduct a careful neurologic and physical examination of the patient and establish a flow sheet for vital signs. Patients who abuse stimulants, especially I.V. stimulants, are at risk for numerous medical complications that can ultimately be more problematic than the intoxication, such as endocarditis, tetanus, hepatitis, abscesses, acquired immunodeficiency syndrome (AIDS),

TRIAGE APPROACH TO DRUG ABUSE

While awaiting laboratory analysis of a drug sample, the clinician can use the chart below to help determine the drug of abuse. A darkened circle indicates that the sign

	STIMULANTS	PHEN-CYCLIDINE	OPIOID OVERDOSE	OPIOID WITHDRAWAL
Autonomic signs				
Hypertension	●	●		
Hypotension				
Tachycardia	●	●		
Hyperthermia	●	●		●
Hypothermia				
Nausea and vomiting	●	●		●
Neurologic signs				
Dilated pupils	●			●
Pinpoint pupils			●	
Nystagmus		●		
Hyperreflexia	●	●		
Hyporeflexia				
Ataxia		●		
Psychological symptoms				
Hallucinations	●	●		
Delusions	●	●		

stroke, intracranial hemorrhage, heart attack, fibrillation, respiratory arrest, and aspiration (Schuckit, 1989).

Laboratory studies

No laboratory tests, other than a toxicology screen, are helpful in diagnosing stimulant intoxication. However, medical complications

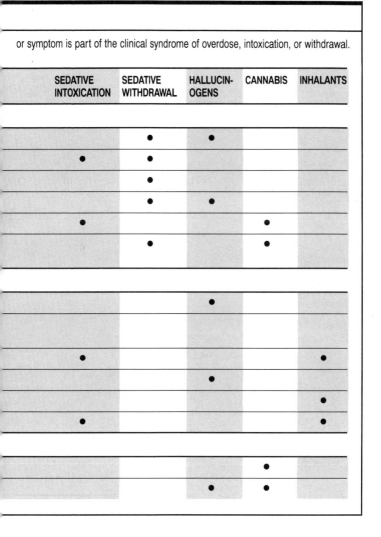

or symptom is part of the clinical syndrome of overdose, intoxication, or withdrawal.

	SEDATIVE INTOXICATION	SEDATIVE WITHDRAWAL	HALLUCIN-OGENS	CANNABIS	INHALANTS
		•	•		
	•	•			
		•			
		•	•		
	•			•	
		•		•	
			•		
	•				•
			•		
					•
	•				•
				•	
			•	•	

that can occur secondary to acute intoxication may warrant such tests, depending on the patient's signs and symptoms.

Differential diagnosis

The differential diagnosis of stimulant abuse must exclude mania, schizophrenia, and phencyclidine intoxication. A toxicology screen is the most effective way to differentiate stimulant intoxication from these other causes; 10 ml of blood and 50 ml of urine are sufficient to carry out appropriate laboratory tests. Recognize, however, that patients with schizophrenia and mania may also abuse stimulants and other drugs, necessitating a dual diagnosis.

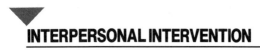

INTERPERSONAL INTERVENTION

Schuckit (1989) recommends placing the patient in a quiet room, away from the general traffic of the emergency department (ED). If the patient is paranoid, avoid a confined setting, which will make him feel threatened, and maintain a comfortable distance between you. Carefully explain all procedures to the patient in detail. Don't touch him without permission, and try to avoid any sudden movements that may disturb him. Reassure the patient that the effects of the stimulant will subside. Because the patient should not be left alone, try to involve family members or friends who can join the session to provide further reassurance.

PHARMACOLOGIC INTERVENTION

If interpersonal interventions fail to relieve the patient's agitation and anxiety, a benzodiazepine, such as diazepam (Valium) 10 mg P.O. or 5 mg I.V. or lorazepam (Ativan) 2 mg P.O. or 2 to 4 mg (0.05 mg/kg) I.M., can be administered. If the patient does not respond to the benzodiazepine or is delusional, extremely agitated, or combative, a high-potency neuroleptic, such as thiothixene (Navane) 10 mg I.M. or 20 mg concentrate or haloperidol (Haldol) 5 mg I.M. or 10 mg concentrate, can be given every 30 to 60 minutes. Low-potency neuroleptics, such as thioridazine (Mellaril) or chlorpromazine (Thorazine), may precipitate an anticholinergic crisis if the patient has ingested a contaminant or unreported anticholinergic substance (see Chapter 16, Psychotropic Drug Reactions). To facilitate excretion of the stimulant, administer ammonium chloride (500 mg P.O. every 3 to 4 hours) with the goal of acidifying the patient's urine below a pH of 6.6 (Schuckit, 1989).

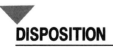

EDUCATIONAL INTERVENTION

Patient education for drug abuse should cover the following:

• Inform the patient and family of the serious medical complications that can result from drug abuse. In particular, warn I.V. drug abusers about the risks of overdose and AIDS.

• Make the patient aware of available rehabilitation programs and self-help groups, and try to dissuade him from trying to "kick the habit" without help because this approach is rarely successful.

• Discuss the importance of ongoing psychiatric treatment in addition to a rehabilitation program if the patient suffers from schizophrenia, depression, or manic episodes. Outline the biological causes of the illness, and emphasize the benefits of and necessity for psychotropic medications. Explain that stimulants can worsen schizophrenic and manic symptoms. If the patient has a major depressive disorder, inform him of the positive prognosis with antidepressant medication.

• Refer a patient with a severe personality disorder for ongoing psychotherapy and rehabilitation treatment, and explain the necessity of psychotherapy to the patient's family (many patients with personality disorders resist psychiatric treatment). Emphasize that the patient, especially a younger patient, is unlikely to "grow out of this phase" and that the severity of the disorder merits ongoing professional intervention.

• Assess the family's role, if any, in the patient's addiction. Family conflicts may precipitate drug abuse. Point out the relationship between family dynamics and drug abuse, and, if appropriate, recommend family therapy. Chaotic and dysfunctional families cannot provide the encouragement and emotional support needed to sustain the patient in ongoing rehabilitation and treatment.

DISPOSITION

With appropriate intervention, stimulant intoxication can be attenuated in the emergency department. Don't discharge the patient, however, until you have completed a thorough drug history and discussed the benefits of a drug rehabilitation program. Schedule the patient for a follow-up appointment the next day with a psychiatrist or a member of a rehabilitation program. When possible, ask the patient's family and friends to encourage his participation in treatment and to help ensure that he does not resume drug use. Caution them that the patient may experience depression, insomnia, and an intense craving for the stimulant.

Consider hospitalizing the patient if he:
• experiences a delusional state that does not remit.
• has a multisubstance abuse problem and requires detoxification from another substance.
• cannot rely on family members or another support system.
• experiences persistent autonomic hyperactivity despite adequate treatment.
• has protracted cognitive impairment.
• has serious associated medical problems.
• has suicidal ideation after discontinuing the stimulant.

Stimulant withdrawal produces an intense craving for the drug, along with depression that can create a suicide risk. Severity of symptoms depends on the potency of the stimulant; I.V. and free-based stimulants cause an especially intense "crash." No detoxification regimen is available for stimulants. Usually, after several nights of sleep, the dysphoria resolves and the suicidal ideation remits. Clinical management involves observing the patient to prevent self-harm and to provide an opportunity for sleep and mood recovery. The clinician should evaluate the patient after sleep to ensure that symptoms of depression and suicidal ideation have disappeared. Occasionally, the suicidal preoccupation may be severe enough to warrant hospitalization. A patient undergoing an acute post-stimulant depression is at high risk for relapse and should be considered a candidate for inpatient rehabilitation. Such a patient may come to the emergency department seeking a sedative-hypnotic to relieve the symptoms (see "Drug-Seeking Behavior" in Chapter 15, Difficult Situations).

MEDICOLEGAL CONSIDERATIONS

Do not discharge a patient who is intoxicated or in acute withdrawal. Make every effort to stabilize him, including hospitalization. If a patient is released prematurely, the emergency service could be held liable for any subsequent harm he causes.

IDENTIFYING THE PROBLEM: PHENCYCLIDINE ABUSE

Phencyclidine (PCP) intoxication commonly presents a confusing clinical picture, with diverse psychological, physiologic, and behavioral effects. Persons can become extremely violent when intoxicated with this drug. Readily absorbed by mouth, smoking, or snorting, PCP is often sold as or is a frequent contaminant of marijuana, lysergic acid diethylamide, cocaine, and amphetamines (Walker, 1983). Its effects usually last 3 to 4 hours but can persist for several days. Consider PCP intoxication a medical emergency, at least until you determine whether the patient's serum drug levels are rising, falling, or stable. No withdrawal syndrome occurs.

Mental status findings
Primary mental status findings include calmness (to the point of sleep), agitation, hostility, disorientation, emotional lability, a sense of slowing of time, "out of body" feelings, belligerence, assaultiveness, unpredictability, impaired judgment, hallucinations, and paranoid ideation.

Physical findings
The physical examination is important for differentiating PCP intoxication from other types. Medical complications — vomiting (with the risk of aspiration), seizures, and extreme hypertension — make the physical evaluation essential to treatment. Establish a flow sheet, record the patient's vital signs at regular intervals, and monitor the patient for laryngeal stridor or respiratory depression. Clinical signs and symptoms usually correlate with dose and blood level (see *Signs and symptoms of phencyclidine intoxication,* page 62).

Laboratory studies
Other than toxicology screens, no routine laboratory tests can aid in diagnosing PCP intoxication. However, based on the physical and

SIGNS AND SYMPTOMS OF PHENCYCLIDINE INTOXICATION

Signs and symptoms of phencyclidine intoxication depend on the amount of drug the patient has ingested and the serum levels produced. Be aware, however, that dosage calibration is nonexistent in drug activity that occurs "on the streets." Also keep in mind that you may need to begin treatment before serum levels are obtained. If ingestion occurred within a few hours of your contact with the patient, be alert to signs of increasing serum levels. An apparently mildly intoxicated patient, left unattended, can soon become gravely distressed and die.

AMOUNT INGESTED	SERUM LEVELS	SIGNS AND SYMPTOMS
1 to 5 mg	10 to 70 ng/ml	Vertical and horizontal nystagmus, dysarthria, ataxia, loss of pain response, drooling, nausea, mild pulse rate and blood pressure elevation, hyperacusis
5 to 20 mg	70 to 200 ng/ml	Catatonia; rigidity, myoclonus; nonresponsiveness to pain, touch, and proprioception; neck spasms; excessive secretions; fever; elevated pulse rate and blood pressure; hyperreflexia
20 mg	> 200 ng/ml	Unresponsiveness to stimuli, pupils fixed and dilated, hypertension, convulsion, death secondary to cardiovascular causes

Source: Weiss, 1983.

neurologic examination and the patient's history, laboratory tests may be clinically indicated.

Differential diagnosis

The differential diagnosis of PCP intoxication includes the effects of other psychoactive substances, such as amphetamines and hallucinogens, as well as head trauma, schizophrenia, delirium, mania, and cerebrovascular accident (Daghestani and Schnoll, 1989). Ataxia, nystagmus, and undilated pupils help rule out stimulant and hallucinogen toxicity. Hyperreflexia and hypertension suggest PCP abuse rather than sedatives or hypnotics. Schizophrenia and mania can usually be ruled out or established based on the patient's history. Closely examine the patient for head trauma and cardiovascular illness.

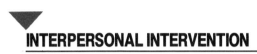

INTERPERSONAL INTERVENTION

Because of the poor judgment of the PCP-intoxicated patient, protective supervision in a nonstimulating environment is essential. In contrast to the approach used for other intoxications, staff members should avoid "talking down" a patient who has taken PCP because it may further agitate him. If possible, obtain a psychiatric and drug use history, including drugs taken, duration of use, time of last dose, and previous adverse reactions. Staff members should carefully search the patient's belongings for drugs or paraphernalia, which can be analyzed to assist in making the diagnosis. (If the patient is lucid, seek his consent first.) Avoid using restraints, if possible, because the patient is at risk for muscle tissue breakdown, which can lead to acute renal failure.

PHARMACOLOGIC INTERVENTION

Pharmacologic treatment of PCP intoxication is complex and should be planned in collaboration with a knowledgeable internist or emergency medicine physician. Treatment for PCP agitation includes the following:

For mild agitation, tension, anxiety, and excitement, administer diazepam 10 to 30 mg P.O. Lorazepam 2 to 4 mg (0.05 mg/kg) I.M. may be used as an alternative in uncooperative patients.

For severe agitation and excitement, with hallucinations, delusions, and bizarre behavior, consider haloperidol 5 mg I.M. or 10 mg concentrate P.O., thiothixene 10 mg I.M. or 20 mg concentrate P.O., or loxapine (Loxitane) 10 mg I.M. or 25 mg concentrate P.O. given every 30 to 60 minutes.

PCP is retained by body fluids, and its metabolism and excretion are influenced by pH levels in urine and gastric acid. Thus, PCP psychosis or delirium can last up to a week, with a waxing and waning of symptoms that reflect excretion into and reabsorption from the stomach, and a principal goal of treatment is to enhance excretion.

If the patient is comatose, administer ammonium chloride 2.75 mEq/kg dissolved in 60 ml of saline solution every 6 hours through a nasogastric tube until the urine pH is less than 5.5. Continuous gastric suctioning is recommended to recover large amounts of PCP left in the stomach.

For a noncomatose patient, urine acidification is accomplished by an I.V. infusion of vitamin C (ascorbic acid) at a rate of 2 g in 500 ml of water every 6 hours (Daghestani and Schnoll, 1989). To ensure an accurate dosage, check the urine pH two to four times a day. When the pH is below 5.0, diuresis can be forced, using furosemide (Lasix) 20 to 40 mg I.V. (Daghestani and Schnoll, 1989). When a diuretic is used, monitor serum electrolytes and administer potassium supplements when necessary.

Urine acidification should continue for at least 1 week; recommended doses are ammonium chloride 500 mg P.O. four times daily and ascorbic acid 1 g P.O. three times daily (Daghestani and Schnoll, 1989). Acidification is contraindicated in patients with severe liver disease and those with renal insufficiency. (See *Complications and treatment of phencyclidine overdose* for additional information.)

▼
EDUCATIONAL INTERVENTION

Educational interventions for PCP abuse are similar to those for stimulant abuse (see page 59).

▼
DISPOSITION

Because of the serious behavioral and medical complications of PCP intoxication, the patient should be admitted for close observation. During hospitalization, a comprehensive drug and psychiatric history should be taken and plans instituted to transfer the patient to a drug treatment program.

COMPLICATIONS AND TREATMENT OF PHENCYCLIDINE OVERDOSE

COMPLICATION	TREATMENT
Seizure and status epilepticus	No medication for a single seizure. For repeated seizures or status epilepticus, give diazepam (Valium) 10 to 20 mg I.V.
Hypertension	Use hydralazine (Apresoline) or phentolamine (Regitine) I.V. infusion 2 to 5 mg over 5 to 10 minutes.
Hyperthermia	Use a cooling blanket
Opisthotonos and acute dystonia	Usually resolves as serum drug levels decrease. If the problem persists, diazepam 2 to 10 mg I.V. is usually effective.
Cardiac arrhythmia	Cardiology consultation
Rhabdomyolysis, myoglobinuria, acute renal failure	Nephrology consultation

Source: Daghestani and Schnoll, 1989, pp. 1213-1214. Adapted with permission of the publisher.

▼

MEDICOLEGAL CONSIDERATIONS

Medicolegal considerations for PCP abuse are similar to those for stimulant abuse (see page 60).

▼

IDENTIFYING THE PROBLEM: OPIOID OVERDOSE

Opioid overdose – from opiates, such as heroin and morphine, and synthetic opioids, such as meperidine (Demerol) and oxycodone (Roxicodone) – is a life-threatening emergency that requires treatment by an experienced internist or emergency medicine physician. Most patients are found in a semicomatose or comatose condition, with recent evidence of I.V. injection, such as a needle in the arm or nearby, or oral ingestion, such as an empty prescription bottle (Schuckit, 1989).

Mental status findings
Because most patients are comatose and need immediate treatment, a complete mental status examination is not indicated.

Physical findings
Characteristic physical findings include decreased respiration; blue lips; blue or pale skin; pinpoint pupils (if brain damage has occurred, usually secondary to anoxia, pupils may be dilated; meperidine can cause mydriasis); hyperemic nasal mucosa (if the drugs have been snorted); recent needle marks on the arm or elsewhere; gasping, rattling respirations and rales secondary to pulmonary edema; and cardiac arrhythmias or seizures, especially when the overdose is caused by codeine, propoxyphene (Darvon), or meperidine (Schuckit, 1989). Death can occur secondary to pulmonary or cerebral edema.

Laboratory studies
The laboratory evaluation should include electrolyte and serum glucose levels, complete blood count (CBC), hepatic and renal profiles, electrocardiogram, arterial blood gas analysis, drug and alcohol screen, and a computed tomography scan. Occasionally, an electroencephalogram may be necessary to establish the level of brain impairment.

Differential diagnosis
Symptoms of opioid overdose warrant immediate treatment with I.V. naloxone (Narcan). If the patient remains comatose, life-support measures should be instituted while other possible causes of the coma are investigated.

▼ INTERPERSONAL INTERVENTION

Because the patient is unconscious, interpersonal interventions are not warranted.

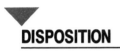

PHARMACOLOGIC INTERVENTION

If the patient does not respond to an opioid antagonist challenge, further treatment is determined by medical complications, such as cardiac arrhythmia or pneumonia (see *Treatment of opioid overdose,* page 68, for guidelines).

EDUCATIONAL INTERVENTION

Educational interventions for opioid overdose are similar to those for stimulant abuse (see page 59).

DISPOSITION

Because of the life-threatening risk of opioid overdose and its potential medical complications, the patient should be hospitalized for further evaluation and treatment.

MEDICOLEGAL CONSIDERATIONS

Medicolegal considerations for opioid overdose are similar to those for stimulant abuse (see page 60).

IDENTIFYING THE PROBLEM: OPIOID WITHDRAWAL

Opioid withdrawal is precipitated by the abrupt cessation of opioid administration after 1 to 2 weeks of continuous use. Administration of a narcotic antagonist, such as naloxone, can also cause opioid withdrawal (*DSM-III-R,* 1987). When heroin or morphine use is discontinued, withdrawal symptoms appear within 6 to 8 hours, peak on the second or third day, and disappear by the 10th day. Meperidine withdrawal begins more quickly, with symptoms appearing within 3 to 4 hours, peaking within 8 to 12 hours, and

---

TREATMENT OF OPIOID OVERDOSE

1. Establish airway.

2. Check pulse rate and initiate advanced cardiac life support, if necessary.

3. Prevent aspiration by positioning the patient on his side or using a tracheal tube with an inflatable cuff.

4. Begin an I.V. infusion with a large-gauge needle.

5. Evaluate for pulmonary edema, blood loss, and cardiac arrhythmias.

6. Administer a narcotic antagonist. Naloxone (Narcan) is the preferred drug, given in doses of 0.4 mg (1 ml) or 0.01 mg/kg I.V. and repeated in 3 to 10 minutes if no reaction occurs. This drug loses its effect in 2 to 3 hours, so the patient in a heroin overdose should be monitored for at least 24 hours and receive methadone (Dolophine) for at least 72 hours.

7. General guidelines for other medical complications include:

(a) blood loss or hypotension—plasma expanders or pressor drugs

(b) pulmonary edema—positive-pressure oxygen, but avoid overoxygenating and decreasing respiratory drive

(c) cardiac arrhythmias—appropriate antiarrhythmic drugs

(d) hypoglycemia—50 ml of 50% glucose

(e) infection—monitor for infection because pneumonia develops in more than 50% of patients with pulmonary edema.

Source: Schuckit, 1989. Adapted with permission of the publisher.

disappearing after 4 to 5 days. Methadone (Dolophine) withdrawal may not begin until 1 to 3 days after the last dose, with symptoms usually dissipating in 10 to 14 days. Withdrawal symptoms for semisynthetic and synthetic opioids are similar to those for heroin. Usually, substances with a short duration of action (such as meperidine) produce intense withdrawal symptoms, whereas substances that are more slowly eliminated (such as codeine) produce milder symptoms.

The amount of opioid that has been ingested can be difficult to determine; for example, about 95% of a "bag" of heroin may consist of adulterants, such as quinine, mannitol, or lactose (Tomb, 1988). Therefore, treatment for opioid withdrawal must be based on objective physical findings rather than on the patient's subjective complaints or statements about opioid habits.

Mental status findings

Most patients are irritable and have a craving for an opioid. Otherwise, no significant mental status findings are associated with opioid withdrawal.

Physical findings

Physical findings—the diagnostic key to recognizing opioid withdrawal—include nausea and vomiting, diarrhea, dilated pupils, muscle aches and pains, insomnia, lacrimation (tearing eyes), flulike weakness, rhinorrhea (running nose), piloerection (goose flesh), sweating, flushing, abdominal pain, increased temperature, yawning, and semen ejaculation.

Laboratory studies

Blood and urine studies are helpful in determining the cause of withdrawal. A physical examination and baseline laboratory studies (CBC, electrolyte and calcium levels, and renal and hepatic profiles) are important because I.V. drug abuse significantly increases the risk for medical complications, including AIDS, hepatitis, endocarditis, pneumonia, and tuberculosis. Staff members must take universal blood and body fluid precautions when handling body fluids of I.V. drug abusers.

Differential diagnosis

The differential diagnosis of opioid withdrawal should exclude sedative-hypnotic and alcohol withdrawal. The clinician can make the diagnosis by testing the patient's blood and urine and by obtaining confirmation of drug use from relatives or friends.

INTERPERSONAL INTERVENTION

A patient in opioid withdrawal is irritable and demanding. To avoid confusion during detoxification, only one clinician should deal directly with the patient. The clinician should explain that he will try to minimize the patient's discomfort although withdrawal symptoms cannot be eliminated. Other staff members should establish a flow sheet of symptom severity.

▼
PHARMACOLOGIC INTERVENTION

A detoxification regimen should be started only when physical signs of withdrawal — such as lacrimation, dilated pupils, rhinorrhea, and piloerection — appear. The two commonly used approaches to opioid detoxification are methadone substitution and withdrawal and clonidine (Catapres) symptom blockade.

Methadone substitution and withdrawal

As described by Weiss and Mirin (1988), methadone treatment should be based on objective physical findings of withdrawal, including a pulse rate 10 beats/minute over baseline (or 90 beats/minute without tachycardia), systolic blood pressure 10 mm Hg over baseline (or 160/95 mm Hg without hypertension), and other signs noted above. Treatment on the first day consists of 5 to 10 mg of methadone every 4 hours as needed for mild to moderate symptoms and 10 to 20 mg every 4 hours as needed for severe symptoms. On the second day, the total amount given during the first 24 hours should be administered in two equally divided doses. On subsequent days, the daily dosage is decreased by 5 mg each day until the patient is no longer receiving methadone.

Clonidine symptom blockade

Clonidine reduces the autonomic symptoms of withdrawal, but the craving, lethargy, insomnia, and restlessness remain. The average dose is 5 mcg/kg of body weight (0.35 mg for a 70-kg patient). The dosage is titrated against symptoms, with the average adult needing 0.3 mg four times daily, or 0.3 to 2 mg/day (Jaffee and Kleber, 1989). After the patient is stabilized, clonidine should be continued for 5 days, with the dosage decreased by 0.2 mg/day. Contraindications include hypotension, use of antihypertensive or antidepressant medication, a history of psychosis or cardiac arrhythmias, and pregnancy. Outpatients should not be given more than three doses of clonidine and must be cautioned about driving during the first several days, because clonidine can be sedating.

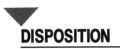

EDUCATIONAL INTERVENTION

Educational interventions for opioid withdrawal are similar to those for stimulant abuse (see page 59).

DISPOSITION

Refer the patient to a methadone maintenance or drug rehabilitation program for further evaluation and treatment. Because opioid withdrawal is not life-threatening, the clinician should not dispense methadone in the emergency setting. Although most patients can be treated in an outpatient setting, hospitalization may be necessary if the patient is addicted to several substances, has a complicating medical illness, or has no family members, friends, or other support system.

MEDICOLEGAL CONSIDERATIONS

Medicolegal considerations for opioid withdrawal are similar to those for stimulant abuse (see page 60).

IDENTIFYING THE PROBLEM: SEDATIVE-HYPNOTIC INTOXICATION

Sedative-hypnotics form a class of drugs that includes benzodiazepines and barbiturates. Sedatives are typically used to control anxiety, whereas hypnotics are used to induce sleep. Sedatives and hypnotics are cross-tolerant and synergistic with alcohol and with each other. Abuse of these drugs in combination with alcohol is one of the most common drug-related causes of morbidity and mortality (National Institute on Drug Abuse, 1987).

Mental status findings

Sedative-hypnotic intoxication is marked by impaired judgment, loquacity, mood lability, dreamlike feelings, and disinhibition of sexual and aggressive feelings.

Physical findings

Slurred speech, uncoordination, unsteady gait, nystagmus on lateral gaze, areflexia, muscle hypotonicity, hypotension, and hypothermia are common physical findings.

Laboratory studies

Baseline values for blood and urine toxicology, CBC, electrolyte levels, and renal and hepatic function should be established at the time of the initial evaluation.

Differential diagnosis

The differential diagnosis of sedative-hypnotic intoxication includes conditions that mimic alcohol intoxication. Therefore, the differential diagnosis must rule out alcohol intoxication (alone or in combination with drugs), as well as hypoglycemia, diabetic ketoacidosis, subdural hematoma, cerebellar ataxia, multiple sclerosis, and Huntington's disease.

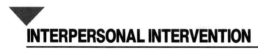

INTERPERSONAL INTERVENTION

Provide clear instructions and information to the patient, identifying yourself as often as necessary and explaining any procedures that must be carried out. The patient usually responds to reassurance and acceptance; thus, friends or relatives can be a useful adjunct to treatment because of the support and familiarity they provide. Place the patient in a well-lighted room under constant supervision, either by staff or family members, to prevent wandering or accidental injury.

Computer =

1. Line over word
2. Copy parts of documents within + across

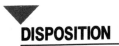

PHARMACOLOGIC INTERVENTION

Management of barbiturate intoxication is a complex medical intervention best left to clinicians who have experience in treating such cases (see *Treatment of sedative overdose,* page 74). Abuse of glutethimide (Doriden) poses a special problem because it is absorbed by adipose tissues and released gradually. Thus, the patient may wake up from a coma only to relapse as more of the drug is released from tissue stores.

EDUCATIONAL INTERVENTION

Some patients indiscriminately abuse prescription sedative-hypnotics in combination with other substances; other patients intentionally abuse sedative-hypnotics as a form of self-medication. In the first case, consider the patient to be evidencing addictive disease, and follow the educational interventions for stimulant abuse on page 59.

Educational interventions differ for the patient attempting self-medication for anxiety, depression, or a psychotic disorder. After eliciting a history of a primary psychiatric disorder, explain to the patient that his symptoms must be controlled under strict medical supervision. Some patients, notably adult children of alcoholics, may overuse sedative-hypnotics to treat anxiety and depression. Because of the risk of addiction, do not administer a benzodiazepine to such patients. Instead, they may benefit from an antidepressant, such as fluoxetine (Prozac), or a nonsedating antianxiety drug, such as buspirone (Buspar). Educational interventions should focus on helping the patient to appreciate the dynamics of his drug abuse and encouraging him to consult a physician for a safer treatment.

DISPOSITION

Barbiturate overdose is a medical emergency. Most patients require admission to a medical intensive care unit for continued evaluation and treatment.

TREATMENT OF SEDATIVE OVERDOSE

1. Establish airway.

2. Evaluate cardiovascular status and initiate advanced cardiac life support, if necessary.

3. Begin I.V. infusion with a large-gauge needle.

4. Establish means to measure urine output.

5. Start gastric lavage if the patient ingested oral medication during the last 4 to 6 hours. Administer 60 ml of castor oil via stomach tube, especially if fat-soluble drugs like glutethimide (Doriden) were taken.

6. Administer 12 to 20 g of activated charcoal suspended in water every 1 to 12 hours over the first 2 days.

7. Check for the possibility of narcotic overdose by giving naloxone (Narcan) 0.4 mg I.M. or I.V.

8. Carry out a thorough neurologic and physical examination.

9. Draw blood for arterial blood gas analysis, general blood tests to evaluate liver and kidney functioning, blood counts, and toxicologic screen.

10. Establish flow sheet for vital signs, level of reflexes, urine output, I.V. fluids.

11. Consider forced diuresis with furosemide (Lasix) 40 to 120 mg, as often as needed to maintain urine output of 250 ml or more per hour. Or I.V. flush with enough saline and water with glucose to maintain urine output at 250 ml or more per hour. This is not needed for patients with stable vital signs or for those who have deep tendon reflexes. Forced diuresis rarely helps for overdoses of chlordiazepoxide (Librium) or diazepam (Valium).

12. Arrange for hemodialysis or peritoneal dialysis for patient in deep coma.

13. Evaluate need for antibiotics. Do not start prophylactically.

14. Do not use a central nervous system stimulant.

Source: Schuckit, 1989. Adapted with permission of the publisher.

MEDICOLEGAL CONSIDERATIONS

Unlike the abuse of illegal drugs, such as cocaine and heroin, abuse of prescription sedative-hypnotics is sometimes perpetuated by duped, misguided, or dishonest physicians. Contributing to prescription abuse – intentionally or unwittingly – increases the patient's risk and magnifies your liability. Before refilling a patient's prescription for a controlled substance, perform a thorough examination, document the indication for treatment, contact the patient's prescribing physician, and limit the refill to a 3-day supply (see "Drug-Seeking Behavior" in Chapter 15, Difficult Situations).

IDENTIFYING THE PROBLEM: SEDATIVE-HYPNOTIC WITHDRAWAL

Left untreated, sedative-hypnotic withdrawal can cause delirium, with significantly increased morbidity and risk for mortality. Additionally, withdrawal can be uncomfortable for the patient because all of its symptoms cannot be suppressed. For these reasons, the patient should be hospitalized.

Withdrawal symptoms do not follow an established pattern. Onset of symptoms correlates with the ingested drug's duration of action. For example, symptoms of pentobarbital (Nembutal) withdrawal begin 12 to 16 hours after the last dose, whereas those of chlordiazepoxide (Librium) withdrawal may not occur until 72 to 96 hours after stopping the drug (see *Sedative-hypnotics and their duration of action,* page 76). Barbiturates usually cause more severe symptoms, but with the advent of high-potency benzodiazepines, such as alprazolam (Xanax) and lorazepam, significant withdrawal symptoms can occur from antianxiety drugs.

Mental status findings
The mental status findings in a patient undergoing withdrawal from a sedative-hypnotic are similar to those of a patient with alcohol withdrawal syndrome: anxiety, a strong desire for the drug, and, in severe cases, hallucinations and delusions.

Physical findings
The physical examination usually reveals tremors, nightmares, insomnia, increased pulse rate and respiration rate, hyperthermia, loss of appetite, nausea and vomiting, postural hypotension, seizures, and delirium. Suspect sedative withdrawal if the patient is agitated, has abnormal autonomic signs, and asks for a sedative.

SEDATIVE-HYPNOTICS AND THEIR DURATION OF ACTION

BENZODIAZEPINES

Long-acting: 20 hours or more
- diazepam (Valium)
- clonazepam (Klonopin)
- chlordiazepoxide (Librium)
- clorazepate (Tranxene)
- flurazepam (Dalmane)
- prazepam (Centrax)

Short-acting: 6 to 19 hours
- alprazolam (Xanax)
- lorazepam (Ativan)
- oxazepam (Serax)
- temazepam (Restoril)

Ultra-short-acting: less than 6 hours
- triazolam (Halcion)

BARBITURATES

Long-acting: 10 to 12 hours
- mephobarbital (Mebaral)
- metharbital (Gemonil)
- phenobarbital (Barbita)

Intermediate-acting: 6 to 8 hours
- amobarbital (Amytal)
- aprobarbital (Alurate)
- butabarbital (Butisol)
- talbutal (Lotusate)

Short-acting: 3 to 4 hours
- pentobarbital (Nembutal)
- secobarbital (Seconal)

Source: Smith et al., 1989. Adapted with permission of the publisher.

Examine the patient carefully; sedative abusers are at risk for many of the same medical problems that occur in opioid abusers, particularly infection and hepatitis.

Laboratory studies

Toxicology screens are indicated to detect multisubstance abuse. A baseline CBC, hepatic and renal profiles, glucose and electrolyte levels, chest X-ray, electrocardiogram (ECG), and blood gas studies can help rule out many other possible causes of delirium.

Differential diagnosis

The differential diagnosis for sedative-hypnotic withdrawal should exclude alcohol withdrawal and other causes of delirium.

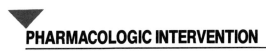

INTERPERSONAL INTERVENTION

Not all patients who are addicted to sedatives are hard-core addicts. Many patients unwittingly become addicted to sedatives prescribed by their physicians, and the addiction may go undiscovered until they are hospitalized for an unrelated medical evaluation or surgery. In this case, the best approach is to explain the addiction to the patient and family. Recommend a psychiatric evaluation to determine whether the patient has an underlying anxiety or sleep disorder. After the evaluation, the patient should be detoxified or referred to a psychiatrist knowledgeable about the specific addiction.

In contrast, hard-core addicts typically exhibit tough, demanding behavior as a defense against feelings of rejection and inadequacy (Renner, 1987), so expect an initial period of defensive hostility. Reassure the patient that you are concerned about him. Because many drug abusers have serious personality disorders, restrict visits to persons of known reliability. Individual and family counseling should start in the hospital, with the goal of enrolling the patient in a long-term program (Renner, 1987). (See also "Drug-Seeking Behavior" in Chapter 15, Difficult Situations.)

PHARMACOLOGIC INTERVENTION

The clinician can choose from several pharmacologic approaches to withdrawing a patient from sedative-hypnotics. One method is effective when the patient's degree of drug use cannot be determined (see *Sedative withdrawal procedure,* page 78). Another

SEDATIVE WITHDRAWAL PROCEDURE

1. Test dose: Administer 200 mg of pentobarbital (Nembutal) orally and assess neurologic changes after 1 hour. The 24-hour pentobarbital requirement is estimated as follows:

PATIENT'S CONDITION 1 HOUR AFTER TEST DOSE	ESTIMATED 24-HOUR PENTOBARBITAL REQUIREMENT (mg)
Asleep, but arousable	None
Drowsy, slurred speech; coarse nystagmus, ataxia, marked intoxication	400 to 600
Comfortable; fine lateral nystagmus is only sign of intoxication	800
No signs of drug effects; perhaps persisting signs of abstinence; no intoxication	1,200 or more

If no signs of a drug effect appear, then repeat the test 3 to 4 hours later using a dose of 300 mg of pentobarbital. No response to the 300-mg dose suggests a habit of more than 1,600 mg/day.

2. Use either pentobarbital or phenobarbital (Barbita) for withdrawal, but phenobarbital has the advantage of few variations of blood barbiturate level. If pentobarbital is used, divide the estimated daily requirement into four equal doses and administer them every 6 hours. If phenobarbital is used, calculate dose at the rate of 30 mg of phenobarbital/100 mg of pentobarbital. Divide the total dose into three equal doses, and administer every 8 hours.

3. Reduce both pentobarbital and phenobarbital at the rate of 10% each day.

4. If the patient is concomitantly dependent on an opiate, barbiturate detoxification should proceed first, to be followed by opiate withdrawal later.

Source: Shader, 1975, pp. 119-120. Adapted with permission of the publisher.

method involves estimating the patient's daily sedative-hypnotic use during the month before treatment (based on the patient's reported history of drug use) and computing a detoxification schedule (see *Phenobarbital conversion from benzodiazepines and sedative-hypnotics*).

PHENOBARBITAL CONVERSION FROM BENZODIAZEPINES AND SEDATIVE-HYPNOTICS

DRUG	DOSE (mg)	PHENOBARBITAL WITHDRAWAL CONVERSION (mg)*
Benzodiazepines		
alprazolam (Xanax)	1	30
chlordiazepoxide (Librium)	25	30
clonazepam (Klonopin)	0.5	30
clorazepate (Tranxene)	15	30
diazepam (Valium)	10	30
flurazepam (Dalmane)	15	30
halazepam (Paxipam)	40	30
lorazepam (Ativan)	1	15
oxazepam (Serax)	10	30
prazepam (Centrax)	10	30
temazepam (Restoril)	15	30
Barbiturates		
amobarbital (Amytal)	100	30
butabarbital (Butisol)	100	30
butalbital (Fiorinal)	50	15
pentobarbital (Nembutal)	100	50
secobarbital (Seconal)	100	30
Glycerols		
meprobamate (Equanil, Miltown)	400	30
Piperidinediones		
glutethimide (Doriden)	250	30

*Withdrawal doses of phenobarbital are sufficient to suppress most withdrawal symptoms but are not the same as therapeutic doses.

Source: Smith et al., 1989. Adapted with permission of the publisher.

Phenobarbital (Barbita) is used to wean patients from sedative-hypnotics because its long half-life prevents a steep decline in blood levels and eases withdrawal. Patients who also abuse alcohol may need a higher dose of phenobarbital. The computed equivalence of phenobarbital is given daily, in three or four divided doses; maximum dosage is 500 mg/day.

After the patient has been stabilized for 2 days, decrease the daily dosage of phenobarbital by 30 mg each day. Before each dose is administered, staff members should check the patient for sustained horizontal nystagmus, slurred speech, and ataxia. If sustained nystagmus is found, the clinician should withhold the scheduled dose. If all three signs are present, the next two doses should be withheld and the total daily dose for the following day cut in half.

If the patient is already in acute withdrawal and in danger of having seizures, the clinician should administer 200 mg of phenobarbital I.M. to stabilize the patient's condition. The withdrawal schedule is then initiated based on one of the protocols described above. If nystagmus or other signs of intoxication develop after the phenobarbital injection, the patient is probably not dependent on sedative-hypnotics.

EDUCATIONAL INTERVENTION

Educational interventions for sedative-hypnotic withdrawal are similar to those for sedative-hypnotic intoxication (see page 73).

DISPOSITION

Because this condition is life-threatening, the clinician should admit the patient for detoxification.

MEDICOLEGAL CONSIDERATIONS

Medicolegal considerations for sedative-hypnotic withdrawal are similar to those for sedative-hypnotic intoxication (see page 74).

▼

IDENTIFYING THE PROBLEM: HALLUCINOGEN INTOXICATION

Hallucinogens comprise two groups of psychoactive substances that differ in chemical structure. The first group, structurally related to 5-hydroxytryptamine, includes lysergic acid diethylamide (LSD), dimethyl-4-phosphoryltryptamine (psilocybin), dimethyltryptamine (DMT), and peyote (mescaline). The second group, created by a series of ring substitutions on amphetamines, includes 2,5-dimethoxy-4-methylamphetamine (DOM or STP), methylene dioxyamphetamine (MDA), methylene dioxymethamphetamine (MDMA), and DOB, a 4-bromo homolog of STP. LSD, mescaline, and the methoxylated amphetamines have a long duration of action (8 to 12 hours), whereas DMT and psilocybin have a shorter duration of action (2 to 6 hours). Hallucinogens cause no known withdrawal symptoms.

Mental status findings

Hallucinogen intoxication is marked by perceptual, emotional, and cognitive changes (Cohen, 1989). With eyes closed, the patient "sees" colorful mobile displays of geometric patterns or complex human or animal forms. Colors become more intense. Fixed objects undulate and flow. The patient has a greater sensitivity to touch and an altered sense of taste and smell, sometimes experiencing synesthesia (an overflow of one sensory modality into another; for instance, the patient "hears" colors or "sees" music). Other perceptual changes include depersonalization, derealization, and body image distortions in which body parts seem to grow, shrink, or disappear.

Emotional alterations range from euphoria, elation, and bliss to tension and anxiety that culminate in a panic attack. The patient may laugh or cry for prolonged periods, usually at inappropriate times.

Cognitive alterations include a loosening of associations with unusual content, illogical and fantasy-laden thought sequences, paranoid grandiosity, and, less commonly, persecutory ideation.

Physical findings
Hallucinogens can cause elevated blood pressure and body temperature, dilated pupils, and hyperactive reflexes.

Laboratory studies
The clinician may order a drug toxicology screen.

Differential diagnosis
The initial diagnosis is usually made by the patient or an accompanying person who verifies that the patient ingested a hallucinogen. Although the clinician typically makes the diagnosis from symptoms (especially the perceptual distortions), the differential diagnosis should rule out anticholinergic, PCP, or cannabis intoxication. A patient on PCP is usually drowsy rather than alert and exhibits such neurologic symptoms as nystagmus and ataxia. Dilated, unreactive pupils are common in anticholinergic intoxication.

▼
INTERPERSONAL INTERVENTION

Interpersonal intervention is crucial when the patient has a "bad trip"—a panic reaction with overwhelming anxiety as a result of the perceptional distortions he is experiencing. The primary intervention involves reassuring the patient that the drug's effects will wear off in several hours. When possible, involve friends and family members, who can help alleviate the patient's anxiety by maintaining a continuous dialogue in a supportive, nonthreatening environment.

▼
PHARMACOLOGIC INTERVENTION

The clinician should try to avoid pharmacologic intervention. If the patient's anxiety becomes overwhelming, he can be given 10 to 30 mg of diazepam P.O. or 2 to 4 mg of lorazepam I.M.

EDUCATIONAL INTERVENTION

That the patient is in an emergency medical setting gives weight to the clinician's educational efforts. Initially, help the patient retain a sense of identity by reassuring him that his hallucinogenic intoxication, although a frightening experience, is nevertheless a drug effect that will subside. Once the patient is free of the drug's effects, focus on preventive measures. He will have already discovered the painful truth that hallucinogen use is far from a benign form of recreation. Remind him that such intoxication can lead to serious injury or death. Encourage the habitual user to participate in drug rehabilitation or counseling. If the patient is a child or adolescent, consider referral to family counseling, since hallucinogen abuse is a form of escape.

DISPOSITION

The effects of a "bad trip" usually remit within several hours, and the patient can be sent home, preferably in the company of family or friends. Arrange an immediate follow-up visit to address the drug problem and to rule out any psychiatric disorders.

Occasionally, a patient enters the ED because of "flashbacks" (recrudescence of symptoms experienced during previous hallucinogenic drug use). This response may appear days, weeks, or months after the last exposure. Treatment of flashbacks is the same as for a hallucinogen-induced panic reaction — reassurance, support, and administration of benzodiazepines to control extreme anxiety.

MEDICOLEGAL CONSIDERATIONS

Although hallucinogen abuse does not carry as high a risk of violent behavior as PCP abuse, violent or self-destructive behavior is possible, especially when hallucinations are frightening. Thus, do not discharge a patient until the drug's effects wear off.

Failure to diagnose hallucinogen abuse — or mistaking it for schizophrenia — is a potential source of liability. Without a coexisting diagnosis of schizophrenia, hallucinogen intoxication does not warrant ongoing antipsychotic drug therapy.

IDENTIFYING THE PROBLEM: CANNABIS INTOXICATION

Cannabis comprises hashish, bhang, marijuana, and purified delta-9-tetrahydrocannabinol (THC). Abusers commonly use cannabis with other substances, particularly alcohol and cocaine. The most common methods of administration are smoking and eating; it is rarely used intravenously. The drug's effects develop 20 to 30 minutes after smoking, longer after oral ingestion.

Mental status findings
A mildly intoxicated patient is euphoric and relaxed. Heightened sexual arousal and decreased social interaction are also typical signs. A patient who has ingested a moderate to heavy amount of cannabis becomes panicky, paranoid, suspicious, and disoriented and may also experience a loss of insight and hallucinations with paranoid delusions.

Physical findings
Physical findings of cannabis intoxication include fine tremor, a slight decrease in body temperature, reduced muscle strength, decreased balance and motor coordination, dry mouth, bloodshot eyes, nausea, and headache. A patient with epilepsy may have seizures.

Laboratory studies
Laboratory studies, such as a toxicology screen, may be ordered to rule out other causes.

Differential diagnosis
The differential diagnosis should exclude intoxication from alcohol, sedative-hypnotics, and opioids.

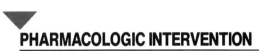

INTERPERSONAL INTERVENTION

The chief intervention for cannabis abuse is reassurance that the symptoms will clear within 4 to 8 hours. Keep the patient in a quiet room, and enlist family and friends to help comfort him.

PHARMACOLOGIC INTERVENTION

A clinician would not usually prescribe psychotropic drugs for a patient with cannabis intoxication. However, if the patient's anxiety and panic become severe, consider administering 10 to 30 mg of diazepam P.O. or 2 to 4 mg of lorazepam I.M. Rarely, paranoia or paranoid delusions warrant neuroleptic medication. Use these agents in small doses for brief periods. Haloperidol 2 to 5 mg P.O. every 24 hours in divided doses is usually adequate. The dosage will rarely need to be increased to more than 20 mg/day.

If a psychotic reaction lasts more than a few days, evaluate the patient for a major psychiatric illness. A patient with cannabis intoxication should not receive an indefinite regimen of neuroleptic medication unless he has an underlying psychiatric illness.

EDUCATIONAL INTERVENTION

Educational interventions for cannabis intoxication are similar to those for hallucinogen intoxication (see page 83).

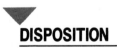

DISPOSITION

A cannabis-intoxicated patient can be managed in the ED, since the reaction remits within 4 to 8 hours. Discharge the patient in the company of a relative or friend, and refer him to a specialist in resolving drug problems. Further psychiatric evaluation is advised to rule out the possibility of coexisting psychopathology. As with hallucinogen abuse, flashbacks can occur with cannabis use. Treatment is similar to that for cannabis intoxication.

▼
MEDICOLEGAL CONSIDERATIONS

Medicolegal considerations for cannabis intoxication are similar to those for hallucinogen intoxication (see page 83).

▼
IDENTIFYING THE PROBLEM: INHALANT ABUSE

Persons who abuse inhalants sniff toluene-containing glue, aerosols, cleaning solutions, nail polish remover, lighter fluids, paint thinner, and other petroleum products. Symptoms of abuse appear within 5 minutes and cease in 1 to 2 hours. An overdose can result in central nervous system depression, cardiac arrhythmias, broncho-spasm, and ventricular fibrillation, any of which can lead to death. Inhalants have no known withdrawal syndromes.

Mental status findings
Mental status findings include belligerence, assaultiveness, apathy, impaired judgment, and impaired social and occupational func-tioning.

Physical findings
Physical findings include dizziness, nystagmus, slurred speech, un-steady gait, depressed reflexes, tremors, blurred vision, diplopia, stupor, coma, rash around the nose and mouth, breath odors, residue on face, hands, and clothing, redness and swelling of the eyes, and irritation of the throat, lungs, and nose. Conduct a thorough physical examination because inhalants can interfere with normal function-ing of most body systems. Major medical problems associated with inhalant abuse include cardiac arrhythmias, hepatitis, renal failure, bone marrow suppression (which can lead to aplastic anemia), impaired pulmonary functioning, and skeletal muscle weakness with muscle destruction (Schuckit, 1989).

Laboratory studies

In addition to a toxicology screen, baseline ECG, CBC, and renal and hepatic studies should be performed because of the potential for serious medical complications.

Differential diagnosis

The differential diagnosis entails ruling out intoxication from alcohol or sedative-hypnotics. Other than results from a toxicology screen, the patient's breath odor or residue on his clothing may provide a clue to inhalant abuse.

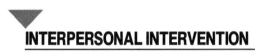

INTERPERSONAL INTERVENTION

Because inhalants have a short duration of action, panic reactions have usually subsided by the time the patient is seen by a clinician. The patient responds favorably to reassurance and support.

PHARMACOLOGIC INTERVENTION

If the patient is in a state of panic on arrival at the ED, the clinician should prescribe 15 to 20 mg of diazepam P.O. or 1 to 2 mg of lorazepam P.O. to control the patient's anxiety.

Chronic, heavy use of inhalants can precipitate withdrawal symptoms within a few hours to several days after cessation of use. These symptoms include tremulousness, tachycardia, disorientation, hallucinations, delusions, agitation, and seizures (Westermyer, 1987). A patient experiencing withdrawal symptoms should be given a long-acting sedative, such as diazepam or phenobarbital (Luminal), in doses sufficient to produce a calm, seizure-free state (Westermyer, 1987). The physician should gradually withdraw the medication over 5 to 10 days.

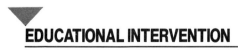

EDUCATIONAL INTERVENTION

Chronic inhalant abusers may have significant cognitive impairment, thus reducing the impact of educational efforts. Impress on the patient the seriousness of this form of substance abuse, and include a younger patient's parents in the discussion (many inhalant abusers are children or adolescents). Inform them that "huffing," even in moderation, can cause brain damage and that its use can hardly be considered recreational. Refer the patient for drug rehabilitation or counseling as indicated.

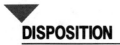

DISPOSITION

If a patient has a complicating medical problem, hospitalization may be warranted. Otherwise, discharge the patient. Schedule an immediate follow-up visit to assess him for underlying psychopathology and to ensure that he is referred to an appropriate treatment program.

MEDICOLEGAL CONSIDERATIONS

Medicolegal considerations for inhalant abuse are similar to those for hallucinogen intoxication (see page 83).

REFERENCES

Cohen, S. "The Hallucinogens," in *Treatments of Psychiatric Disorders: A Task Force Report of the American Psychiatric Association.* Washington, D.C.: American Psychiatric Association, 1989.

Daghestani, A.N., and Schnoll, S.H. "Phencyclidine Abuse and Dependence," in *Treatments of Psychiatric Disorders: A Task Force Report of the American Psychiatric Association.* Washington, D.C.: American Psychiatric Association, 1989.

Diagnostic and Statistical Manual of Mental Disorders, 3rd ed. Washington, D.C.: Amerian Psychiatric Association, 1987.

Gawin, F.H., and Ellinwood, E.H.: "Stimulants," in *Treatments of Psychiatric Disorders: A Task Force Report of the American Psychiatric Association.* Washington, D.C.: American Psychiatric Association, 1989.

Jaffee, J.H., and Kleber, H.D.: "Opioids: General Issues and Detoxification," in *Treatments of Psychiatric Disorders: A Task Force Report of the American Psychiatric Association.* Washington, D.C.: American Psychiatric Association, 1989.

National Institute on Drug Abuse. "Trends in Drug Abuse-Related Hospital Episodes and Medical Examiner Cases for Selected Drugs." Drug Abuse Warning

Network (DAWN) 1976 to 1985, Series H, #3. Rockville, Md.: United States Department of Health and Human Services, 1987.

Renner, J.A. "Drug Addiction," in *Massachusetts General Hospital Handbook of General Hospital Psychiatry*, 2nd ed. Edited by Hackett, T.P., and Cassem, N.H. Littleton, Mass.: PSG Publishing Company, Inc., 1987.

Schuckit, M.A. *Drug and Alcohol Abuse: A Clinical Guide to Diagnosis and Treatment*, 3rd ed. New York: Plenum Medical Book Company, 1989.

Shader, R.I., et al. "Treatment of Dependence on Barbiturates and Sedative-Hypnotics," in *Manual of Psychiatric Therapeutics*. Edited by Shader, R.I. Boston: Little, Brown and Company, 1975.

Smith, D.E., et al. "Barbiturate, Sedative, Hypnotic Agents," in *Treatments of Psychiatric Disorders: A Task Force Report of the American Psychiatric Association*. Washington, D.C.: American Psychiatric Association, 1989.

Tomb, D.A. *Psychiatry for the House Officer*, 3rd ed. Baltimore: Williams and Wilkins, 1988.

Walker, J.I. *Psychiatric Emergencies: Intervention and Resolution*. Philadelphia: J.B. Lippincott, 1983.

Weiss, K.J. "Phencyclidine Intoxication and Abuse," in *New Psychiatric Syndromes: DSM-III and Beyond*. Edited by Akhtar, S. New York: Jason Aronson, 1983.

Weiss, R.D., and Mirin, S.M. "Intoxication and Withdrawal Syndromes," in *Manual of Psychiatric Emergencies*, 2nd ed. Edited by Hyman, S.E. Boston: Little, Brown and Company, 1988.

Westermeyer, J. "The Psychiatrist and Solvent Inhalant Abuse: Recognition, Assessment, and Treatment," *American Journal of Psychiatry* 144(7):903-907, July 1987.

SCHIZOPHRENIA AND MANIA

A patient who suffers from an acute psychosis displays disorganized thinking, distorted perceptions, intensified and unrealistic feelings, and inappropriate behavior (Barsky, 1984). The patient has a substantially impaired ability to perceive and deal with reality. In an acute psychotic state, the patient cannot communicate with or relate to others normally and cannot meet the demands of ordinary life. This chapter reviews the differential diagnosis of and treatment interventions for schizophrenia and mania.

IDENTIFYING THE PROBLEM

Although schizophrenia and mania share many characteristics and typically require similar interventions, the conditions sufficiently differ in onset of symptoms, patient presentation, and mental status findings to warrant separate discussions in these areas.

Schizophrenia
A patient who suffers from schizophrenia has impaired thought content, thought process, perceptions, affect, sense of self and purpose, and interpersonal functioning (*DSM-III-R*, 1987). However,

the psychiatric emergency is usually precipitated when delusions, hallucinations, or disturbed behavior become severe. At times, a patient with milder symptoms – withdrawal, inappropriate or flat affect, impaired personal hygiene, impaired level of functioning, bizarre perceptions or ideas, and disturbed communication – may appear in the emergency department (ED).

Because many patients with schizophrenia appear bizarre, ill-kempt, loud, and agitated, staff members may view them as "weird" or "out of it" and minimize or ignore their problems. ED staff may become uncomfortable in their presence, inadequately evaluate them for underlying medical illness, and provide only superficial psychiatric treatment in order to discharge them as soon as possible. In one reported case, a patient who was initially diagnosed as a homeless, chronic schizophrenic was ultimately found to have severe hypothyroidism (Shader and Greenblatt, 1987).

A clinician cannot make a definitive diagnosis of schizophrenia until the patient exhibits continuous signs of the illness for at least 6 months. Schizophrenia usually begins during adolescence or early adulthood, although it can develop later.

Mania

Manic episodes have an acute onset, with rapid escalation of symptoms over a few days (*DSM-III-R*, 1987). During such episodes, the patient has a considerably impaired ability to function in normal social and work situations. One of the most common complications is substance abuse, which results from impaired judgment. A patient with mania may participate in varied multiple activities (sexual, occupational, political, religious). He may attempt to renew friendships after a lapse of many years, calling old friends in the middle of the night. The manic patient may occasionally dress in flamboyant or bizarre clothing; women may wear several shades of lipstick, heavy makeup, and numerous bracelets and necklaces.

A manic patient does not usually see his behavior as intrusive or demanding. The patient's comments can be inappropriate, perhaps overtly sexual. Because of a remarkable sensitivity to other people's personal vulnerabilities, the patient typically makes unnerving, sarcastic comments about staff members and can quickly exhaust their patience. Once the patient perceives their negative reactions, he becomes louder and more extroverted, usually to the point where force is needed to restrain him.

The condition characteristically develops between ages 20 and 30, although some cases involving patients over age 50 have been reported. Mania occurs most commonly in patients with a bipolar disorder, characterized by a history of mood swings between manic episodes and major depressive episodes.

Mental status findings: Schizophrenia

A patient with schizophrenia has fragmented and bizarre delusions, ranging from persecution delusions (the patient believes that others are spying on, spreading false rumors about, or planning to harm him) to ones of reference, in which objects or other people are given particular or unusual significance (for instance, the patient may be convinced that a television commentator is mocking him). Delusions are also common: the patient may believe that his thoughts are being broadcast from his head to the external world for others to hear or that his thoughts have been inserted into or removed from his mind by some external force (*DSM-III-R,* 1987).

Hallucinations, especially auditory hallucinations, are common in schizophrenic patients. Voices — which the patient perceives as coming from outside his head — may make insulting remarks, speak directly to him, or comment on his behavior. Command hallucinations, in which the patient hears voices that must be obeyed, can sometimes create danger for him or others. A patient may report that "the voice is telling me to kill my wife." Tactile and somatic hallucinations and, less commonly, visual, gustatory, and olfactory hallucinations also occur. As a rule, if a patient complains of non-auditory hallucinations, suspect delirium, alcohol intoxication, drug withdrawal, or other organic mental disorders.

Schizophrenia is also characterized by thought disorder. Loosening of associations, in which ideas shift from one unrelated subject to another, is the most common example. The patient is unaware that the topics are disconnected, and statements that lack a meaningful relationship may be juxtaposed. The severely schizophrenic patient is incoherent.

The patient's affect is either flat or inappropriate. A flat affect is manifested by emotionless expression and monotonous speaking. The patient may also exhibit disturbed psychomotor behavior, becoming completely unaware of his environment. He may maintain rigid postures and resist efforts to be moved; make apparently purposeless and stereotyped excited movements that are not influenced by external stimuli; or assume inappropriate or bizarre postures.

Mental status findings: Mania

The manic patient may be unusually cheerful. His elevated mood, characterized by unceasing and unselective enthusiasm, can have an infectious quality. However, the patient may also be irritable or angry. At other times, the patient's mood may be labile, rapidly changing from elated playfulness to anger and rage.

A manic patient's sense of self-esteem can reach a point of grandiosity and may be delusional. For example, the patient may claim to have a PhD, mention that the President of the United States seeks his advice, or speak of being sent by God to Earth for special missions. As in schizophrenia, a manic patient may experience hallucinations, the content of which is usually consistent with the predominant mood; for example, he may hear God's voice explaining a special mission or persecutory voices.

Other characteristics of mania include a decreased need for sleep (the patient may not sleep for days); rapid, loud, unintelligible speech; distractibility; and flight of ideas (the patient changes abruptly from topic to topic, based on understandable associations, distracting stimuli, or wordplay; in serious cases, the patient becomes severely disorganized and incoherent).

Physical findings: Schizophrenia and mania

Although a physical examination is not helpful in making a diagnosis of schizophrenia or mania, you must conduct a thorough physical evaluation to rule out medical illness as a cause of the patient's psychosis. According to Anderson (1980), the examination should include an assessment of the patient's general appearance and vital signs and an evaluation of the patient's head (for injuries), eyes (for pupil size and presence of nystagmus or exophthalmos), neck (for rigidity or thyroid enlargement), skin (for color and perspiration), hands (for tremor, asterixis, or chorea), and reflexes (for hyperactivity, asymmetry, and the presence of snout and grasp reflexes).

Laboratory studies: Schizophrenia and mania

Laboratory studies are of little value in diagnosing schizophrenia or mania. Nevertheless, a complete blood count, electrolyte level, renal and hepatic profiles, chest X-ray, electrocardiogram, blood gas analysis, and alcohol and drug screens may help rule out medical causes of the psychosis. If the patient is stuporous and lethargic or experiences an acute onset of symptoms, a computed tomography scan and lumbar puncture may detect central nervous system causes of the disorder.

Differential diagnosis: Schizophrenia and mania

Many medical disorders can cause symptoms similar to those of schizophrenia and mania (see *Medical disorders that mimic schizophrenia and mania*). If the patient has delusions, hallucinations, and disorganized thought but is fully oriented, you can usually rule out organic brain syndromes. Additionally, any one of the following features suggests an underlying medical illness: a first psychotic episode after age 40, disorientation, abnormal vital signs, stupor or lethargy (clouded consciousness), visual hallucinations, or illusions (Dubin et al., 1983; Hall et al., 1978).

Perhaps the most difficult differential diagnosis to make in the emergency setting is between mania and paranoid schizophrenia (*DSM-III-R*, 1987). Both manic and schizophrenic patients can be irritable, hypersensitive, and paranoid. However, in contrast to a patient with schizophrenia, the manic patient has a history of discrete recurrent episodes of mania and depression, with a return to normal functioning between episodes. Additionally, catatonic symptoms of schizophrenia—stupor, mutism, negativism, and posturing—are rarely seen in manic patients.

▼ INTERPERSONAL INTERVENTION

Treatment of any patient in a psychiatric emergency is inextricably linked to the initial interview, which not only elicits important diagnostic information but also can be therapeutic. Your primary goal is to gather information about the patient's current illness, psychiatric and medical history, family and occupational history, and drug or alcohol use.

MEDICAL DISORDERS THAT MIMIC SCHIZOPHRENIA AND MANIA

Drug toxicities
- Corticosteroids
- Digitalis
- Disulfiram (Antabuse)
- Isoniazid (Laniazid)
- Levodopa (Dopar)
- Methyldopa (Aldomet)

Endocrine disorders
- Addison's disease
- Cushing's syndrome
- Hyperparathyroidism
- Hypoparathyroidism
- Hypothyroidism

Heavy metal intoxication
- Lead
- Manganese
- Mercury
- Thallium

Infections
- Bacterial meningitis
- Cerebrovascular syphilis
- Delirium secondary to cerebral infection
- Postencephalitic syndrome

Neurologic disorders
- Cerebral neoplasm
- Degenerative diseases of the central nervous system
- Multiple sclerosis
- Normal-pressure hydrocephalus
- Temporal lobe (complex partial) epilepsy

Substance abuse disorders
- Alcohol hallucinosis
- Alcohol-delusional disorder
- Alcohol withdrawal and intoxication
- Amphetamine intoxication
- Barbiturate and similar substance withdrawal
- Drug-induced mania
- Idiosyncratic alcohol intoxication
- Phencyclidine intoxication

(continued)

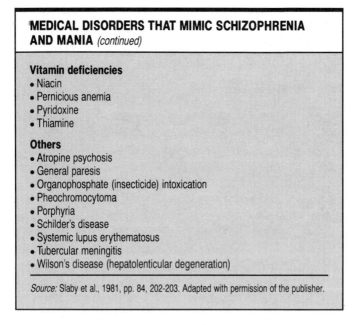

MEDICAL DISORDERS THAT MIMIC SCHIZOPHRENIA AND MANIA *(continued)*

Vitamin deficiencies
- Niacin
- Pernicious anemia
- Pyridoxine
- Thiamine

Others
- Atropine psychosis
- General paresis
- Organophosphate (insecticide) intoxication
- Pheochromocytoma
- Porphyria
- Schilder's disease
- Systemic lupus erythematosus
- Tubercular meningitis
- Wilson's disease (hepatolenticular degeneration)

Source: Slaby et al., 1981, pp. 84, 202-203. Adapted with permission of the publisher.

Conducting the interview: General guidelines

When possible, conduct the interview in a quiet room where you and the patient can sit comfortably. If the interview is conducted after the medical evaluation, remove unnecessary medical equipment, such as intravenous needles, to prevent injury. Always introduce yourself, and address the patient formally (such as "Mr. Jones" or "Ms. Harper") to help restore the patient's dignity. Begin with general questions rather than asking for specific medical details:

"How are you? Can we talk for a little while?"

"Would you like something to eat before we talk?"

"Can I do anything to make you feel more comfortable?"

"Would you like me to contact anyone for you?"

Only after the patient begins to feel comfortable should you start asking about the specifics of his illness. To obtain more detailed information, avoid questions the patient can answer with a simple "Yes" or "No," and try to keep the interview flexible rather than following a rigid format. Also, keep in mind that a psychotic patient, although appearing out of touch with reality, may be partially or fully aware of what is happening around him. Finally, try to refrain from laughing excessively when a patient makes witty remarks; overly friendly or casual responses can cause the patient to react negatively when you resume the interview with a more measured manner (Hanke, 1984).

Establishing empathy

The patient may be reluctant to participate in the interview because of a need to protect his sense of integrity and self-control. To overcome this reluctance, establish emotional contact by empathizing with his feelings. Most psychiatric patients are extremely sensitive and usually unwilling to risk expressing themselves to impatient, irritable, or condescending clinicians. Try to understand the patient's predicament of being in a hospital and not knowing what will happen.

If the patient remains relatively calm but verbally uncooperative or if he appears too anxious, you may choose to drop a particular subject and return to it later in the interview when he is more receptive. Food, a symbol of caring, can also help you develop a rapport with many patients. Offering juice or crackers is appropriate, but avoid hot liquids to prevent injury.

The disorganized, hallucinating, or delusional patient

When interviewing a patient with disorganized thinking, structure the interview by asking straightforward questions. If the patient begins to ramble, indicate that you understand what he is saying and help him organize his thoughts. Unless the patient is paranoid, you can begin to establish rapport through physical contact; for instance, ask for permission to take his blood pressure or feel his forehead.

When a patient has hallucinations and delusions, do not attempt to correct the misperceptions; instead, explore how they are experienced by the patient. Avoid the temptation to use logic to convince the patient that he is wrong. Such an approach makes the patient more defensive.

The unresponsive patient

If a psychotic patient does not respond to questioning, use any available information to make contact with him. Such data may include the patient's words, expressions, appearance, or behavior, as well as your feelings. Make specific comments, such as "I see you are in a bathrobe. I gather you were brought to the hospital unexpectedly."

If the patient is unable or unwilling to provide clinical information, try to talk with a relative or friend or with clinicians who have previously treated him. When possible, obtain the patient's consent to contact these persons, but remember that life-threatening situations, such as suicidal or homicidal behavior, take precedence over confidentiality; then, you have a responsibility to contact family or friends regardless of whether the patient has given permission. In such cases, carefully document the reasons for breaching confidentiality (see Chapter 2, Medicolegal Considerations).

The paranoid patient

Of all psychiatric patients, the paranoid patient is the most difficult to evaluate, perhaps because he can instill fear in the clinician (Perry, 1976). If the patient displays threatening behavior, try to conceal your fear initially. The patient may quickly sense your discomfort and become frightened, which could lead to a violent episode. At times, however, you may have to acknowledge your fear by saying, "The way you are looking at me is scary, like you are on the verge of striking out. I won't be able to give you my full attention if I am afraid." Remaining professionally confident and maintaining eye contact usually reassures the patient. To reduce anxiety—yours and the patient's—conduct the interview with the door open or with other staff members present.

Use tact when interviewing a paranoid patient, who is easily humiliated and made to feel guilty for actions and thoughts. Don't challenge his beliefs or question distorted notions. If you try to determine what is real and what is not, the patient may regard you as a prosecutor putting him on trial, and he may become more defensive and argumentative.

If an angry patient begins a tirade of accusations about being mistreated, you may have to interrupt by asking, "How can I help you?" When interviewing such a patient, maintain a safe professional distance; don't become overly friendly or engage in joke telling. Be advised that a highly paranoid patient can make you feel defensive and foolish by twisting the meaning of your words, making it impossible to sustain any direction to the interview. Under these circumstances, alter the course of the interview by telling the patient he is making you uncomfortable and ask him to discuss his reasons for doing so. If meaningful contact cannot be made, terminate the interview.

The catatonic patient

Patients in a catatonic stupor have a substantially decreased ability to react to the environment, and they make few spontaneous movements (*DSM-III-R*, 1987). Administering amobarbital (Amytal) can markedly facilitate the interview, although the procedure is time-consuming (see *Using amobarbital during a patient interview,* page 100). As an alternative, lorazepam (Ativan) 2 mg I.M. or I.V. followed by a maintenance dose of oral lorazepam 1 mg twice daily can produce dramatic and sustained improvement in patients with catatonia (Salam and Kilzieh, 1988).

Mutism — usually an angry response that symbolizes an attempt by the patient to control the environment — may be concomitant with catatonia or occur alone. Although medical and neurologic disorders have been reported as causes of mutism, it is usually a sign of mental illness. The first step in psychiatric management of mutism is to indicate to the patient that you expect verbal responses to your questions. If the patient continues to remain silent, try to determine what the patient may be communicating through his silence. Never express a sense of futility by repeatedly asking questions and receiving no reply. If you cannot persuade the patient to talk, obtain diagnostic information from family members or friends, and admit the patient to the psychiatric unit for evaluation and treatment.

Terminating the interview

Although you may be under considerable pressure to work rapidly, all psychiatric patients deserve sufficient time to express their feelings and concerns. Conclude each interview by summarizing your understanding of the patient's problem, your recommendations for further care, and your reasons for making such recommendations.

USING AMOBARBITAL DURING A PATIENT INTERVIEW

1. Have the patient recline.

2. Explain that the medication should make the patient relax and feel like talking.

3. Insert a narrow-bore scalp-vein needle into the forearm or hand.

4. Begin injecting a 5% solution of amobarbital (Amytal) – 500 mg dissolved in 10 ml of sterile water – at a rate no faster than 1 ml/minute (50 mg/minute) to prevent sleep or sudden respiratory depression.

5. Interview:
   (a) With a verbal patient, begin with neutral topics, gradually approaching areas of trauma, guilt, and possible repression.
   (b) With a mute patient, continue to suggest that soon the patient will feel like talking. Prompting with known facts about the patient's life may also help.

6. Continue the infusion until the patient shows sustained rapid lateral nystagmus or drowsiness. Slight slurring of speech is common; the sedation threshold is usually reached at a dose between 150 mg (3 ml) and 350 mg (7 ml), but can be as little as 75 mg (1.5 ml) in an elderly patient or one with organic illness. Prompts to talk should have their strongest effect at this point.

7. To maintain the level of narcosis, continue the infusion at the rate of 0.5 to 1.0 ml every 5 minutes.

8. Conduct the interview as you would any other psychiatric interview, but with several caveats:
   (a) Approach affect-laden or traumatic material gradually and then work over it again and again to recover forgotten details, attendant feelings, and the patient's current reactions to them.
   (b) In the mute or verbally inhibited patient, do not concentrate on traumatic topics (such as murderous rage towards someone) to prevent the development of panic after the interview.

9. Terminate the interview when enough material has been produced (about 30 minutes for a mute patient), or when therapeutic goals have been reached (sometimes an hour or more). Have the patient recline for an additional 15 minutes until he can walk with close supervision.

Source: Perry and Jacobs, 1982, p. 559. Adapted with permission of the publisher.

PHARMACOLOGIC INTERVENTION

Rapid tranquilization (RT) is usually safe and effective for controlling agitated, potentially assaultive, or overtly violent patients (Dubin et al., 1986). RT is accomplished by administering a standard dose of neuroleptic medication over 30 to 60 minutes to treat severe agitation, anxiety, tension, hyperactivity, or excitement. Most patients respond to RT within 30 to 90 minutes.

RT by itself is not a complete treatment. The clinician should use RT as an adjunct to verbal intervention and as part of an overall clinical approach that involves treating the patient in a humane, concerned manner. Core psychotic symptoms, such as delusions, hallucinations, and disorganized thought, do not respond to a few doses of medication; weeks of neuroleptic therapy are required before these symptoms begin to subside. Before using RT, clearly explain to the patient why the medication is needed (for instance, "You seem to be restless and nervous. This medication will make you feel calm and help stop the voices you are hearing"). Using such terms as "violent," "out of control," "crazy thoughts," or "strange behavior" as reasons for medication will agitate the patient. Furthermore, most patients do not like to be sedated and should be told that the medication will not induce sleep.

Route of administration

Although many clinicians prefer I.M. injection, oral concentrate is an effective alternative and should be considered the method of choice (Dubin et al., 1986). However, never threaten the patient if he refuses the concentrate; instead, be patient and persistent. Use an injection only after several efforts to administer the concentrate have failed. Under no circumstances should you offer a drink containing the concentrate without the patient's knowledge. Contrary to the belief that patients may be too agitated and uncooperative to take concentrate, most will cooperate with an oral dosing regimen (Dubin et al., 1985).

For some patients—those with lowered cardiac output who cannot absorb I.M. medication, those incapable of taking oral medication, and those with extensive tissue damage, such as from major burns—I.V. administration may be necessary.

Dosage

One to three doses of neuroleptic medication given every 30 to 60 minutes is usually sufficient to control a psychotic, agitated patient. Symptoms begin to subside within 20 to 30 minutes of the first dose. Used in equivalent doses, all neuroleptic agents are equally effective. If the patient reports or his record indicates that a particular medication has been helpful, this can be the drug of choice. In general, a patient should not receive more than six doses in 24 hours, although no correlation has yet been found between the number of required doses and the patient's size, age, sex, diagnosis, previous history, or medical illness. Thus, the clinician must determine the total number of doses empirically.

Alternative drugs

Benzodiazepines can be used as an alternative to neuroleptic medication, especially in treating mania (Dubin, 1988). Although both lorazepam and clonazepam (Klonopin) have been proven effective in controlling symptoms of mania, lorazepam in I.M. form is rapidly and efficiently absorbed.

A suggested protocol for lorazepam is 2 to 4 mg (0.05 mg/kg) every 2 hours as needed. Lorazepam has no established overall maximum dose and must be titrated according to the patient's condition. Side effects include ataxia, respiratory depression, and mild orthostatic blood pressure changes. Withdrawal symptoms and behavioral disinhibition do not develop in patients given lorazepam during RT.

Extrapyramidal side effects

Selection of a neuroleptic drug depends on the side effects that the clinician wants to induce (sedation with low-potency drugs) or avoid (hypotension with low-potency drugs or extrapyramidal side effects [EPS] with high-potency drugs). As a general rule, do not administer low-potency neuroleptic drugs to patients with cardiac illness, delirium, or suicidal tendencies (Hyman and Arana, 1986).

EPS develops in less than 10% of patients within the first 24 hours of RT (Dubin et al., 1986). EPS is not dose related and can occur after one dose. The most common EPS is a dystonic reaction: involuntary turning or twisting movements produced by massive and sustained muscle contractions (Mason and Granacher, 1980).

Dystonia usually involves muscles of the back, neck, and mouth. The patient may extend his back (opisthotonos) or arch his head severely backward (retrocollis) or sideways (torticollis) (Hyman and Arana, 1986). His eyes may be pulled upward in a painful manner (oculogyric crisis). At times, the patient may complain of "thickness" of his tongue or difficulty swallowing. The most serious form of dystonia is laryngospasm. This contraction of the muscles of the larynx can compromise the airway and lead to severe respiratory distress. Although laryngospasm is rare, be alert to its possible occurrence. Because a dystonic reaction develops suddenly and produces bizarre behavior, it can be misdiagnosed as a conversion disorder (an alternation or loss of physical functioning that suggests a physical disorder but is actually an expression of a psychological conflict).

Another EPS that is commonly misdiagnosed is akathisia, which can be mistaken for a psychotic decompensation. A patient with akathisia is uncomfortably restless and finds relief only by pacing. He may describe himself as "unable to relax," "tense," "all wound up like a spring," "irritable," or "jumping out of my skin" (Van Putten and Marder, 1987). Severe akathisia can lead to rapid psychotic decompensation; in its most serious manifestation, it may lead to suicide or homicide (Van Putten and Marder, 1987). In the emergency setting, akathisia may occur in the following situations:

• After two or three doses of RT, a patient's behavior appears to worsen.

• A patient calms down after RT but becomes agitated and psychotic several hours later.

• A patient who has been taking his medication is brought into the ED because of an apparent relapse.

Treatment for acute dystonia and akathisia is 2 mg of benztropine (Cogentin) or 50 mg of diphenhydramine (Benadryl) I.M. or I.V. These doses can be repeated every 5 minutes for up to three doses. Most patients experience dramatic relief within 1 to 3 minutes after injection, although a small number may not respond. In these cases, diazepam (Valium) 5 to 10 mg I.V. or lorazepam 2 to 4 mg (0.05 mg/kg) I.V. or I.M. may help. In an agitated patient with a severe thought disorder, the clinician may not be able to distinguish akathisia from psychotic excitement. One way to resolve this is to treat the patient for akathisia; if he responds positively to benztropine or diphenhydramine, the diagnosis of akathisia can be made.

Whether patients should be given prophylactic treatment for EPS during RT remains unclear. In the first 24 hours after RT, few EPS appear, and most patients do not need antiparkinsonian agents. However, the clinician should prescribe prophylactic antiparkinsonian drugs for patients who have a previous history of EPS, who are reluctant to take medication for fear of EPS, or who are paranoid and in whom EPS may lead to noncompliance.

If a patient receives RT in the ED and is then admitted to the hospital, the clinician should order benztropine or diphenhydramine as needed. Dystonia or akathisia may occur several hours after RT. If the patient is discharged after RT, he should be given several 2-mg benztropine tablets to take if he develops dystonia or akathisia.

Other side effects

Although EPS are the most common side effects of RT, less common side effects — neuroleptic malignant syndrome, hypotension, and seizures — may occur.

Neuroleptic malignant syndrome is an extremely serious idiosyncratic response; its hallmark symptoms are autonomic instability with hyperthermia, hypertension, and "lead-pipe" rigidity (Lazarus et al., 1989). This reaction occurs in approximately 1% of patients receiving antipsychotic medication. To date, this phenomenon has not occurred in patients undergoing RT (Lazarus et al., 1989). Do not be deterred from using RT because of concerns about neuroleptic malignant syndrome, but be aware of its risk factors, which include young age (20 to 40 years), chronic psychosis, male sex, dehydration, malnourishment, and placement in poorly ventilated rooms or in restraints (Mueller, 1985).

Hypotension is a common risk from low-potency antipsychotic agents. If hypotension occurs, the patient should be kept in a supine or reverse Trendelenberg position and given I.V. fluids for hypovolemia. Administer alpha-adrenergic agonist drugs only, such as levarterenol (Levophed) or metaraminol (Aramine). Mixed alpha- and beta- or beta-adrenergic drugs, such as isoproterenol (Isuprel) and epinepherine (Adrenalin), can further reduce blood pressure (Bassuck et al., 1984).

Antipsychotic medication during RT rarely causes seizures; they have been reported in only two patients receiving low-potency neuroleptic agents (Dubin and Feld, 1989).

No cases of sudden death from RT have been reported. The cardiovascular safety of antipsychotic medication has been demonstrated repeatedly (Donlon et al., 1979; Clinton et al., 1987), particularly in patients with severe, unstable cardiovascular illness (Dubin et al., 1986). Other potential side effects (tardive dyskinesia, sexual dysfunction, endocrine disturbances, and photosensitivity) usually develop from long-term use of neuroleptic drugs and are not of concern in RT.

▼
EDUCATIONAL INTERVENTION

The psychiatric emergency setting is not ideal for educating a schizophrenic patient about the illness and its treatment. However, a psychoeducational intervention to prevent relapses should be included as part of most clinical contacts. Discuss the following points with the patient and family members:

• Schizophrenia is a mental illness that usually does not resolve by itself.

• Staying well requires a long-term commitment to treatment.

• Persons suffering from schizophrenia are sensitive to stress.

• Neuroleptic medication can alleviate some symptoms, such as hallucinations, fear, and agitation.

• Neuroleptic medication can cause side effects, such as tardive dyskinesia and extrapyramidal symptoms.

• Noncompliance with the drug regimen can cause relapse.

• Knowing the early signs of relapse can help avert rehospitalization. (The patient may stop taking his medication, miss work, ignore personal hygiene, stop eating or eat more than usual, or become withdrawn and begin talking to himself.)

The manic patient's unique psychological defenses – denial, grandiosity, projections, and distortion – make an educational agenda in the emergency setting difficult for the clinician. Nevertheless, you should cover the following points with the patient and family members:

- Prevention—through strict compliance with the prescribed medication regimen—is the best treatment.
- Recognize the early signs of relapse, such as decreased need for sleep, excessive energy, rapid talking, unrealistic business or personal plans, or indiscreet behavior.
- Use medication conscientiously.
- Staying well requires a long-term commitment to treatment.

DISPOSITION

Many patients who experience an acute manic or schizophrenic episode can be treated and discharged from the ED. As part of the disposition planning, you should contact the patient's family members or friends if they did not arrive with the patient. Relatives and friends can usually provide a history of the patient's response to and compliance with medication therapy, which is essential for determining effective treatment. Furthermore, they may help convince the patient to accept a treatment recommendation, especially if inpatient treatment is needed.

Before discharging a patient, arrange a follow-up appointment for the next day, either as an outpatient or in a partial (day) hospital. Ensure that the patient is accompanied by a family member or friend, who should observe him for the next 24 hours and take him to the scheduled appointment. If the patient received neuroleptic medication in the ED or was given a prescription for neuroleptic medication, several 2-mg tablets of benztropine should also be prescribed. Discuss the possibility of EPS with the patient and family members. Tell them to report any side effects to the prescribing physician, and instruct family members to give the benztropine to the patient immediately if dystonia, akathisia, or laryngospasm develops (the last condition also warrants an immediate trip to the nearest ED).

A psychotic patient should be hospitalized if he:
- shows no improvement after interpersonal and pharmacologic interventions.
- improves but remains psychotic and has no family members or friends willing or able to stay with him.
- poses a threat to himself or others.

• has a condition of unknown severity.

• requires high doses of medication or needs medication frequently.

▼
MEDICOLEGAL CONSIDERATIONS

The clinician must consider the medicolegal consequences of treating schizophrenic or manic patients.

Schizophrenia

Competent patients can legally refuse medication, hospitalization, and other interventions unless they are demonstrably dangerous or under a court order for treatment. Because a patient has been brought in by the police does not lessen this right. In addition, failure to obtain informed consent because you suspect the patient will refuse treatment can be considered a breach of duty.

The essential criterion for committing a schizophrenic patient is *dangerousness,* the definition of which (usually found on the commitment form) varies from state to state. Clinically, dangerousness encompasses self-destructive and outwardly aggressive behavior and an inability to care for one's basic needs. When a psychotic but nondangerous patient is also incompetent, apply for commitment, shifting the burden of disposition to the court.

Because clinicians can be held legally responsible for a patient's dangerous behavior, you must protect known or unknown potential victims by hospitalizing the patient, starting civil commitment procedures, or warning any potential victims identified by the patient. If the patient is not committable and has threatened unknown persons, contact the hospital lawyer to avoid any legal complications, and consider filing a report with the police. Clinicians can also be held legally accountable for harm to persons or property caused by a patient who was prematurely released, even if the harm occurs several months after discharge. Emergency personnel must be mindful of this liability when releasing any patient.

Mania

The disposition of a patient with mania can be difficult. The patient may not believe that he needs treatment, refusing to cooperate with attempted treatment interventions and even refusing to remain in the ED for evaluation. Many hypomanic patients have impaired judgment yet retain formal aspects of competency. You should respect the patient's right to refuse treatment up to the point at which civil commitment criteria are met. Most states permit emergency detention of a competent but self-destructive manic patient (for example, a patient who walks naked on a highway or picks fights in a rough neighborhood). Obviously, an irritable or enraged manic patient who has threatened or harmed others should be detained.

An aggressive and paranoid manic patient may divulge plans to harm specific or unnamed persons. As with the schizophrenic patient, you may have a responsibility to warn potential victims or notify the police. By threatening others, the patient has probably also met the criteria for civil commitment, which you have a duty to pursue. A patient in an early stage of mania may be marginally psychotic, not demonstrably dangerous, and not committable. If you suggest voluntary hospitalization and the patient refuses, make every effort to form a treatment alliance (an agreement between the patient and the clinician that specifies treatment goals). Carefully document plans for follow-up care and, if possible, release the patient to another party, agency, or institution.

REFERENCES

Anderson, W.H. "The Physical Examination in Office Practice," *American Journal of Psychiatry* 137(10):1188-1192, October 1980.

Barsky, A. "Acute Psychoses," in *Emergency Psychiatry: Concepts, Methods, and Practices.* Edited by Bassuck, E.L., and Birk, A.W. New York: Plenum Press, 1984.

Bassuck, E.L., et al. "General Principles of Pharmacologic Management in the Emergency Setting," in *Emergency Psychiatry: Concepts, Methods, and Practices.* Edited by Bassuck, E.L., and Birk, A.W. New York: Plenum Press, 1984.

Clinton, J.E., et al. "Haloperidol for Sedation of Disruptive Emergency Patients," *Annual of Emergency Medicine* 16(3):319-322, March 1987.

Diagnostic and Statistical Manual of Mental Disorders, 3rd ed., revised. Washington, D.C.: American Psychiatric Association, 1987.

Donlon, P.T., et al. "Cardiovascular Safety of Rapid Treatment with Intramuscular Haloperidol," *American Journal of Psychiatry* 136(2):233-234, February 1979.

Dubin, W.R. "Rapid Tranquilization: Antipsychotics or Benzodiazepines," *Journal of Clinical Psychiatry* 49(suppl):5-11, December 1988.

Dubin, W.R., and Feld, J.A. "Rapid Tranquilization of the Violent Patient," *American Journal of Emergency Medicine* 7(3):313-320, May 1989.

Dubin, W.R., and Weiss, K.J. "Emergency Psychiatry," in *Psychiatry,* volume 2. Edited by Michels, R., et al. Philadelphia: J.B. Lippincott Company, 1985.

Dubin, W.R., et al. "Organic Brain Syndrome: The Psychiatric Imposter," *JAMA* 249(1):60-62, January 1983.

Dubin, W.R., et al. "Pharmacotherapy of Psychiatric Emergencies," *Journal of Clinical Psychopharmacology* 6(4):210-222, August 1986.

Dubin, W.R., et al. "Rapid Tranquilization: The Efficacy of Oral Concentrate," *Journal of Clinical Psychiatry* 46(11):475-478, November 1985.

Hall, R.C.W., et al. "Physical Illness Presenting as Psychiatric Disease," *Archives of General Psychiatry* 35:1315-1320, 1978.

Hanke, N. *Handbook of Emergency Psychiatry.* Lexington, Mass.: The Collamore Press, 1984.

Hyman, S.E., and Arana, G.W. *Handbook of Psychiatric Drug Therapy.* Boston: Little, Brown and Company, 1986.

Lazarus, A., et al. *The Neuroleptic Malignant Syndrome and Related Conditions.* Washington, D.C.: American Psychiatric Press, Inc., 1989.

Lazarus, A., et al. "Rapid Tranquilization with Neuroleptics: Neurologic Concerns," *Clinical Neuropharmacology* 12:303-311, 1989.

Mason, A.S., and Granacher, R.P. *Clinical Handbook of Antipsychotic Drug Therapy.* New York: Brunner/Mazel, 1980.

Mueller, P.S. "Neuroleptic Malignant Syndrome," *Psychosomatics* 26(8):654-662, August 1985.

Perry, J.C., and Jacobs, D.L. "Overview: Clinical Applications of the Amytal Interview in Psychiatric Emergency Settings," *American Journal of Psychiatry* 139(5):552-559, May 1982.

Perry, S. "Acute Psychotic States," in *Psychiatric Emergencies.* Edited by Glick, R.T., et al. New York: Grune and Stratton, 1976.

Salam, S.A., and Kilzieh, N. "Lorazepam Treatment of Psychogenic Catatonia: An Update," *Journal of Clinical Psychiatry* 49(suppl):16-21, December 1988.

Shader, R.I., and Greenblatt, D.J. "Back to Basics – Diagnosis Before Treatment: Hopelessness, Hypothyroidism, Aging, and Lithium," Journal of Clinical Psychopharmacology 7(6):375-376, December 1987.

Slaby, A.E., et al. *Handbook of Psychiatric Emergencies,* 2nd ed. New Hyde Park, N.Y.: Medical Examination Publishing Co., Inc., 1981.

Van Putten, T., and Marder, S.R. "Behavioral Toxicity of Antipsychotic Drugs," *Journal of Clinical Psychiatry* 48/49(suppl):13-19, September 1987.

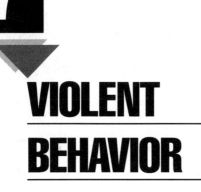

VIOLENT BEHAVIOR

Managing a violent patient can be one of the most challenging tasks facing the clinician, whose interventions can have life-saving consequences. Adding to the complexity of treating such patients is the usual need to make clinical decisions based on relatively incomplete psychological assessments and vague histories. Furthermore, violent patients evoke in clinicians feelings of fear, anger, and rejection and thoughts of retaliation. Despite these obstacles, you can successfully treat a violent patient if you approach him in an objective, systematic manner.

IDENTIFYING THE PROBLEM

Violent behavior occurs in all diagnostic categories; your immediate task in an emergency setting is to contain it. Evaluation, diagnosis, and disposition can occur only after the patient is controlled. Violence rarely occurs spontaneously and is usually preceded by a prodrome characterized by the following features:

■ **Increasing anxiety and tension.** This may be marked by a clenched jaw or fist, rigid posture, or fixed facial expression. At times, the anxiety and tension are manifested by somatic symptoms, such as shortness of breath, rapid pulse, or sweating.

■ **Verbal stridency.** When the patient becomes verbally abusive and profane, the risk of patient mismanagement increases because clinical judgment can be clouded if you personalize the abuse and react emotionally.

■ **Hyperactivity.** This is the most important predictor of imminent violence. Because the hyperactive patient is at highest risk for violence, you should evaluate him immediately. Never ignore a patient's motor hyperactivity.

Many potentially violent patients make verbal threats. To avoid overreacting, note the patient's behavior as well as the threat. Although the patient is hostile and angry, his behavior may indicate that an assault is not imminent. For example, a patient who puts his hands in his pockets, crosses his arms, or assumes some other nonthreatening position usually poses no danger, even if he is making loud verbal threats. In contrast, a patient who refuses to cooperate with any of your requests poses a high risk for violence.

When evaluating a patient for violent behavior, you may be tempted to avoid asking questions about the patient's past, since knowledge of previous assaults can create unbearable anxiety in the interviewer. Nevertheless, patients must be questioned about all types of past violence, with attention to the frequency, severity, and recentness of the violent acts (Monahan, 1982). Crucial information includes the history of arrests and convictions for violent crimes; juvenile court involvement; mental hospitalizations for dangerous behavior; violence at home toward spouse, child, or self; and reported violence toward others (Monahan, 1982). Assessing previous use of alcohol and drugs and ownership of weapons is also critical for determining the patient's risk for violent behavior (Lion et al., 1968).

Mental status findings

In the emergency setting, most patient violence results from a psychotic episode. Mental status findings that suggest psychosis include psychomotor agitation, hallucinations, delusions, and disturbed thought.

Physical findings

Evaluating a patient in the middle of a violent episode is usually not possible. However, you should conduct a physical examination as soon as feasible to rule out medical causes of violent behavior, such as alcohol or drug intoxication or withdrawal. Be alert for nystagmus; hyperreflexia; elevated blood pressure, pulse rate, and temperature; dilated pupils; and slurred speech.

Laboratory studies

A toxicology screen can detect drug and alcohol abuse. A complete blood count, electrolyte level, renal and hepatic screens, blood gas analysis, and electrocardiogram can help detect an underlying medical cause. Additional studies depend on the patient's history and results of the physical examination.

Differential diagnosis

The differential diagnosis is important to rule out delirium as a cause of violence, because a mistaken diagnosis can result in increased morbidity and risk of mortality. Hypoglycemia, chronic obstructive pulmonary disease, renal failure, pneumonia, cardiac disease, and alcohol or substance abuse can also cause violent behavior. Suspect delirium if the patient has a sudden onset of symptoms, is over age 40 and has no previous psychiatric history, appears disoriented, has abnormal vital signs, and experiences visual hallucinations and illusions (see *Differential diagnosis of violent patients*).

Organic mental disorders

Of special concern is a patient with an organic mental syndrome secondary to substance abuse or withdrawal. Because alcohol and barbiturate intoxication cause behavioral disinhibition, a patient in withdrawal may react unpredictably. A patient who is intoxicated from cocaine, amphetamines, or phencyclidine or who has alcohol withdrawal syndrome can be agitated and delusional and may become violent.

Schizophrenia and mania

A patient with paranoid schizophrenia is at high risk for violence. He may respond to delusions of persecution by retaliating against

DIFFERENTIAL DIAGNOSIS OF VIOLENT PATIENTS

Delirium
- Sudden onset
- Disorientation
- Waxing and waning of symptoms
- Visual hallucinations
- Illusions
- Known medical illness
- Patient on medication for medical illness
- No previous psychiatric history necessary

Alcohol or drug intoxication or withdrawal
- Tremor
- Pupillary changes
- Hyperreflexia
- Nystagmus
- Slurred speech
- Ataxia
- Autonomic hyperactivity
- History of drug or alcohol use
- Physical signs of drug use (needle tracks, nasal septum erosion)
- Requests for controlled substances

Personality disorder
- Absence of hallucinations, delusions, disorganized thought
- Orientation intact
- History of impulsive behaviors, including self-mutilation, suicide gestures or attempts, sexual promiscuity, drug abuse, shoplifting, excessive spending
- History of antisocial behavior, including stealing, drug use, destroying property, frequent physical fights, engaging in an illegal occupation

Schizophrenia or mania
- Gradual onset
- Hallucinations
- Delusions, especially persecutory
- Disorganized thought
- Orientation intact
- History of psychiatric illness

the presumed source of the harassment or obey command hallucinations that order him to act violently. In some cases, the patient may be so disorganized that his violence relates to purposeless, excited motor activity (Tardiff, 1989). A manic patient can become violent if you deny or ignore his demands.

Personality disorders

Patients with character disorders, especially antisocial or borderline personalities, also pose a significant threat of violence (see Chapter 15, Difficult Situations). When such patients are intoxicated by alcohol or drugs, they have little concern for property or personal rights. They are also emotionally immature, impulsive, and hostile and have poor judgment and a low tolerance for stress (Lion, 1972).

INTERPERSONAL INTERVENTION

When interviewing a violent or potentially violent patient, take precautions to minimize physical risks. Stay at least an arm's length away from the patient at all times. Neither you nor the patient should feel trapped in the interview room, and you both should have immediate access to the door. To reduce anxiety, either leave the door open or, if you still feel uncertain of the patient's potential for violence, conduct the interview in the hallway. Remove from the room any objects that can be used as weapons, such as heavy ashtrays, pictures, or chairs. If possible, have soft pillows available to use as shields and a panic button to summon additional staff immediately if you are attacked. Additionally, Tardiff (1989) advises clinicians to remove their eyeglasses, neckties, necklaces, and earrings.

Some patients attempt to coerce or intimidate a clinician into admitting them to the hospital or giving them controlled drugs. Never reject or fulfill such requests immediately. Instead, calmly listen to the patient's story to gather a history for evaluating mental status. Rejecting a patient's request—especially without adequately exploring it—can precipitate a violent reaction. If you later decide to discharge a patient who has requested admission, summon staff members before informing the patient of the treatment plan.

Handling a patient with a weapon

The greatest threat to the clinician comes from a violent patient who carries a weapon. Because increasing numbers of patients carry weapons, many hospitals now have metal detectors. In addition to guns and knives, however, the patient may use his fists or any available weapon – a chair, an ashtray, a telephone, or a crutch.

If the patient admits to carrying a weapon, recognize it as a symbol of defense against feelings of helplessness and passivity (Salamon, 1976). Immediately requesting that the patient give up the weapon may heighten these feelings and further exacerbate his agitation, although you should notify hospital security so that they can be available if the patient tries to use the weapon. If the patient volunteers to surrender the weapon, do not accept it directly. Instead, ask the patient to put it on the floor or table so you can take it at the end of the interview.

If the patient threatens you with a weapon, try not to exacerbate his feelings of helplessness, impotence, and shame. The most effective approach is to speak to the patient in a calm manner and admit fear and anxiety (Dubin et al., 1988), saying "I would like to help you, but I feel threatened and frightened by the weapon. I have difficulty listening to you under these circumstances." This may be sufficient to disarm the patient. Never make verbal counterthreats or become physically aggressive; these responses can trigger assaults.

Understanding the dynamics of violence

Aggression usually represents a defensive stance against overwhelming feelings of helplessness and fragility (Lion, 1972). The patient's hypermasculine behavior is commonly an overreaction to his strong sense of impotence, uselessness, and inability to control the environment (Bach-y-Rita et al., 1971). These feelings are usually aroused before an episode of physical violence. Staff members who feel threatened may respond in an authoritarian, counteraggressive manner. As a result, the patient's feelings of helplessness and impotence are intensified, and a violent confrontation ensues. Therefore, your first step is to understand your own reactions to the violent patient.

Some clinicians respond to violent behavior with fear, anxiety, or frustration. A common reaction is that the violent patient belongs in jail or is an untreatable psychopath or alcoholic (Lion and Pasternak, 1973). The clinician who feels this way can fail to gather historical data that may explain the patient's previous violent acts. Most clinicians feel vulnerable in the presence of a violent patient, fearing that the patient may become aggressive if his expectations are not fulfilled. A clinician may also feel angry and helpless because the patient's behavior reflects badly on the clinician's professional abilities or because the patient may do something for which the clinician will be held liable (Lion and Pasternak, 1973). A clinician who feels terrorized may project his fears onto the patient and perceive the patient as being more hostile and threatening than he may be. Thus, expectation of violence may cause it.

The clinician must also confront profanity and verbal abuse. A clinician who is the target of verbal stridency may personalize the abuse, which creates a negative emotional reaction that can cloud clinical judgment and jeopardize decision making. Verbal abuse, like violent behavior, is a defense against feelings of helplessness and passivity and must be viewed in the context of the patient's overall predicament — being evaluated and treated by a staff of strangers who sometimes make disparaging remarks and perhaps being handcuffed or restrained in an emergency department or hospital against his will. The appropriate response to verbal abuse is to proceed with the clinical evaluation in an effort to understand the causes of the patient's symptoms. A harsh and punitive response to verbal tirades augments the patient's feelings of helplessness, increasing the chance of violence.

Using verbal intervention
Most violent patients are terrified of losing control and welcome therapeutic efforts to prevent them from acting out (Lion et al., 1972). You can reduce the patient's anxiety and fear by maintaining a humane, respectful manner. Empathetic, verbal intervention is the most effective method of calming an agitated, fearful, panicky patient. A patient who is treated with honesty, dignity, and respect is more likely to believe that you are going to help him. Once a patient feels hope, you can establish a therapeutic rapport.

Address the patient formally, using Mr., Mrs., or Ms., to convey respect. Begin the interview with benign topics, such as the patient's age, address, and schooling, and avoid a hasty discussion of the reasons for the patient's violent behavior (Lion, 1972). If the patient does not respond to the initial interventions, do not feel rejected or rebuffed, even when the patient is hostile. With gentle persistence, encourage the patient to talk, which provides an outlet for his tension. Most disturbed patients are relieved to know that someone recognizes their need for help.

Establishing empathy

Because of the stress and fatigue of working in an emergency setting, you may have difficulty establishing empathy for a violent patient. Yet a sensitive awareness of his emotional turmoil can provide insight into his behavior. Carefully phrased comments — such as "I can understand how you feel" or "It must be terribly upsetting to be brought into an emergency department and not know what is happening or going to happen" — may stimulate conversation. You can further empathize with the patient by trying to view the situation from his perspective. Can you imagine what hearing voices or having thoughts that you can't control must be like? To be in handcuffs or restraints, lying on your back, with no one around but strangers? To be so anxious and tense that you feel as if you are going to explode?

You can also begin to establish rapport by offering the patient food or drink, which usually calms a hostile patient and confirms that you are concerned. A patient is unlikely to assault a therapist who has just fed him. Offer only cold drinks, such as orange juice, to potentially violent patients because hot drinks can be used as weapons.

Addressing the patient's affect

Efforts to calm a patient through rationalization and logic only increase his agitation. In contrast, encouraging the patient to talk about angry feelings can help him confront reality by demonstrating that violent fantasies and wishes, unlike violent behavior, are not destructive. Many psychotic patients cannot differentiate between fantasies and actual behavior.

Setting limits

Most patients tend to respond to a clinician's expectations of self-control, and a violent patient's behavior may worsen if the clinician does not set certain limits at the outset of the interview. Thus, you should clearly tell the patient that violence is unacceptable and describe the consequences (such as restraints or seclusion) if violence occurs.

A clinician can set limits directly or indirectly (Thackery, 1987). Using the direct approach, you would clearly specify the required behavior in positive terms ("do this") rather than negative ones ("don't do that"). The direct approach is most effective for a confused or disorganized patient with a psychotic or organic disorder, although you may need to refocus and reorient the patient by repeating your directives.

Using the indirect approach, you would attempt to decrease the patient's will to resist by forcing him to choose from several acceptable alternatives (for example, "You have a choice. You can either take this medication and go to the interview room to talk, or, if you feel out of control, you can sit in a seclusion room until you feel less anxious"). Because opposing a single directive is easier than focusing simultaneously on alternatives, the patient's resistance is reduced. Most patients choose the desired alternative. The indirect approach is most effective for a patient who is not confused or severely disorganized; thus, he can differentiate internal stimuli (hallucinations and delusions) from external stimuli (your voice and suggestions).

PHARMACOLOGIC INTERVENTION

If a patient does not respond to interpersonal intervention, rapid tranquilization (RT) can effectively attenuate agitation and excitement. Although anxiety, tension, and hyperactivity are dramatically reduced by RT, hallucinations and delusions remit only after 10 days or more of standard neuroleptic medication. RT is typically safe and effective for treating violence secondary to schizophrenia, mania, delirium, and drug and alcohol intoxication and withdrawal (Dubin and Feld, 1989). If the clinician can determine the cause of the violence, drug intervention should be as specific as possible, especially in cases of alcohol and drug intoxication and withdrawal (see *Drug treatment of the violent patient*). Dystonia and akathisia are the most common side effects of RT. Treatment for these adverse effects includes 25 to 50 mg of diphenhydramine (Benedryl) or 1 to 2 mg of benztropine mesylate (Cogentin) I.M. (See Chapter 6, Schizophrenia and Mania, and Chapter 16, Psychotropic Drug Re-

DRUG TREATMENT OF THE VIOLENT PATIENT

CAUSE OF VIOLENT BEHAVIOR	DRUG INTERVENTION
Schizophrenia, mania, or other psychosis	thiothixene (Navane) 10 mg I.M. or 20 mg concentrate
	haloperidol (Haldol) 5 mg I.M. or 10 mg concentrate
	loxapine (Loxitane) 10 mg I.M. or 25 mg concentrate (All doses given at 30 to 60 minute intervals. One-half dose for medically ill or older patients.)
Personality disorder	lorazepam (Ativan) 1 to 2 mg P.O. every 1 to 2 hours or 2 to 4 mg I.M. (0.05 mg/kg) every 1 to 2 hours
Alcohol withdrawal states	For agitation, tremors, or change in vital signs: chlordiazepoxide (Librium) 25 to 50 mg P.O. every 4 to 6 hours
	For elderly patients or patients with liver disease: lorazepam 2 mg P.O. every 2 hours
	For extreme agitation: lorazepam 2 to 4 mg I.M. every hour or rapid tranquilization* of patient not controlled with benzodiazepines
Cocaine and amphetamine intoxication	For mild to moderate agitation: diazepam (Valium), 10 mg P.O. every 8 hours
	For severe agitation: thiothixene 20 mg concentrate or 10 mg I.M.; haloperidol 10 mg concentrate or 5 mg I.M.
Phencyclidine intoxication	For hyperactivity, mild agitation, tension, anxiety, excitement: diazepam 10 to 30 mg P.O., or lorazepam 2 to 4 mg (0.05 mg/kg)
	For severe agitation and excitement with hallucinations, delusions, bizarre behavior: haloperidol 5 to 10 mg I.M. every 30 to 60 minutes

*Rapid tranquilization in alcohol withdrawal states is for severe agitation and behavioral control. The actual treatment of withdrawal is with a cross-tolerant medication.

actions, for extensive discussions of RT side effects and their treatment.)

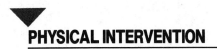

PHYSICAL INTERVENTION

When interpersonal and pharmacologic interventions fail to control the violent patient, the clinician must resort to physical intervention. Alert hospital security and other staff members before violent behavior escalates, using a code name, such as "Dr. Armstrong," to avoid disturbing the patient. Controlling the patient is more difficult if you wait until he is on the verge of violence before summoning help.

The arrival of security guards conveys to the patient that his violent impulses will be controlled and also helps allay the fears of the staff (Lion et al., 1972). However, the patient should not be made to feel that security personnel are there to challenge his masculinity or threaten his passivity (Salamon, 1976). Ideally, security guards should be visible but appear nonthreatening, and in most cases they need not be brought into the interview room. When they arrive, a staff member should tell them why they were called, and you should direct personnel accordingly. Relinquish control only if another staff member is more skilled and experienced in managing such situations.

Restraints
Although few patients require it, restraining is an integral part of treatment, usually when a clinician cannot contain the patient's behavior (Lenefsky et al., 1978). The clinician must never threaten a patient with restraints but, when necessary, should use them immediately and without belligerence (Bell and Palmer, 1981). All staff members should receive appropriate instruction so that patients can be restrained as smoothly and efficiently as possible (see *Guidelines for using restraints*).

According to the American Psychiatric Association (Task Force Report #22, 1985), restraints may be used to:
• prevent imminent harm to the patient or staff members when other means of control are ineffective or inappropriate

GUIDELINES FOR USING RESTRAINTS

1. At least four persons should be used to restrain the patient, while a fifth staff member controls the patient's head and prevents him from biting. At no time should only one or two persons try to restrain a patient. Leather restraints are the safest and surest type of restraint.

2. Explain to the patient why he is being restrained. Give the patient a few seconds to comply, but do not negotiate. At a prearranged signal, the team grabs the patient and brings him to the floor in a backward motion without injuring him. The team applies restraints, then moves the patient to the seclusion room after uniformly lifting the patient.

3. A staff member should always be visible to reassure the patient who is being restrained. This helps alleviate the patient's feeling of helplessness.

4. Restrain the patient with legs spread-eagled and one arm restrained to the side and the other arm restrained over the patient's head.

5. Remove all dangerous objects from the patient, including rings, shoes, matches, pens, and pencils.

6. Place restraints so that intravenous fluids can be given if necessary.

7. Raise the patient's head slightly to decrease his feelings of vulnerability and to reduce the possibility of aspiration.

8. Check the restraints every 5 minutes to ensure safety and comfort.

9. After the patient is in restraints, begin treatment using verbal intervention or rapid tranquilization.

10. Remove one restraint at a time at 5-minute intervals until the patient has only two restraints on. Remove both of these restraints at the same time. Do not leave only one limb in restraints.

Source: Dubin and Weiss, 1985, p. 9. Adapted with permission of the publisher.

- prevent serious disruption of treatment or significant damage to property
- decrease patient stimulation
- respond to a patient's request for them.

Preventive aggressive devices (PADS) are a less restrictive method of controlling patients with a history of aggressive behavior and can be considered as an alternative to restraints. (Van Rybroek et al., 1987). Wrist PADS allow the patient to eat, smoke, and protect himself from falls; ankle PADS allow the patient to walk and participate in unit activities.

Restraints are contraindicated in a patient with an unstable medical condition from infection, cardiac illness, disorders of body temperature regulation, metabolic illness, or orthopedic problems. A patient with delirium or dementia may experience a worsening of symptoms secondary to the sensory deprivations of restraints (Task Force Report #22, 1985).

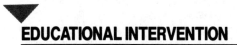

EDUCATIONAL INTERVENTION

Patient education depends on the cause of the violent behavior. If the violence is caused by medical illness, reassure the patient and family that future violence is unlikely once the underlying condition is corrected. If violence occurs secondary to a psychosis, such as schizophrenia or mania, teach the family to recognize the early symptoms of relapse so that treatment can be initiated in time to avert a violent episode. Also discuss the potential triggers of violence, when known, and acquaint family members with the mental health commitment laws in case the patient's condition worsens and he refuses to accept treatment.

Inform a patient whose violence results from alcohol or drug abuse that intoxication or withdrawal syndromes do not relieve him of responsibility for his behavior. Educate the patient and family about the long-term medical consequences of drug and alcohol abuse. Warn an abuser of intravenous drugs about the risk of acquired immunodeficiency syndrome. Also inform a patient with a personality disorder that his condition does not relieve him of responsibility for his behavior and that he can be held legally liable for his actions.

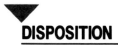

DISPOSITION

In most instances, a violent patient must be detained so that you can determine the cause of the violence, establish the diagnosis, initiate treatment, and assess risks for future violence. Most violent patients meet the criteria for hospitalization (see Chapter 6, Schizophrenia and Mania).

Occasionally, you may discharge a patient if the violence is secondary to an alcohol or drug intoxication that has been treated in the emergency setting. Refer the patient to a rehabilitation program because the violence can become problematic if the patient resumes substance abuse.

If the police bring in a violent patient who has a personality disorder, carefully evaluate him for psychosis and substance abuse. If you find no evidence of these problems, release the patient to legal authorities.

▼
MEDICOLEGAL CONSIDERATIONS

Managing a violent patient amounts to a balancing act for the clinician, who must weigh the patient's right to freedom and autonomy against the community's right to protection from violence (Tardiff, 1989). The clinician must distinguish between using seclusion, restraints, or medication for his own convenience and using them for the benefit of the patient and society. Four legal issues of particular relevance to the violent patient and the clinician are informed consent, refusal of treatment, dangerousness, and duty to warn or protect intended victims.

Informed consent
The doctrine of informed consent recognizes the patient's right to control what is happening to his body and mind. To meet the criteria for obtaining informed consent, a clinician must explain all treatment alternatives and risks to the patient, who must then agree to be treated.

According to Tardiff (1989), treating a violent patient may supercede the need for informed consent if:
• the patient's problem constitutes a psychiatric emergency that does not allow adequate time for informed consent (for instance, when a patient is violent or imminently violent toward others)
• the patient is deemed incompetent because he cannot understand information given to him about his illness and treatment benefits, risks, and alternatives (in nonemergency situations, family members should make decisions about treatment and provide their consent;

in an emergency, the clinician can make decisions about treatment without obtaining consent from the patient or family).

Refusal of treatment

A clinician must honor the patient's legal right to refuse medication or any other treatment – unless the patient is incompetent or becomes a danger to himself or others. In certain states, the reason for refusal must be determined and carefully documented by the clinician. Procedures for administering medication to an incompetent patient against his will differ among jurisdictions. Some jurisdictions provide for an independent review by mental health professionals not involved with the patient's daily treatment; others provide for a judicial review to determine the patient's competency (Tardiff, 1989).

If the patient is competent, the clinician must determine why the patient refuses medication. Possible reasons include insufficient information about the drugs, cultural or religious beliefs, and pressure from family or friends.

Dangerousness

A patient's degree of dangerousness is determined by several factors, including recent acts of violence, evidence of intoxication, mental status findings, the reliability of statements by family members or friends, and the clinician's judgment. Mental illness is only one cause of violent behavior, however. If the clinician determines that the patient's actions were not caused by a psychosis (a requisite concept in commitment laws), the patient should be relegated to the criminal justice system. You may release such a patient to the police.

Duty to warn or protect

Clinicians are justifiably concerned about the consequences of committing an involuntary patient or releasing a patient who is unpredictably dangerous. A related concern is the clinician's duty to warn the intended victim of a violent patient. This issue becomes especially complex in an emergency setting because the clinician usually does not have an ongoing relationship with the patient. In most states, the clinician's duty is to protect, but not necessarily to warn, intended victims.

RISK FACTORS FOR VIOLENCE

- Signs of alcohol or drug use
- Agitation, anger, disorganized behavior
- Poor compliance during the interview
- A detailed or planned threat of violence
- Available means for inflicting injury, such as ownership of a weapon
- History of violence
- History of childhood physical abuse
- Presence of organic disorder
- Presence of psychotic psychopathology, especially paranoid delusion or command hallucinations
- Presence of organic, borderline, or antisocial personality disorder
- Belonging to a demographic group with an increased prevalence of violence: young, male, lower socioeconomic group

Source: Tardiff, 1989. Adapted with permission of the publisher.

To fulfill the requirement of the duty to protect, the clinician must gather comprehensive information to decide whether the patient has a short-term potential for violence (see *Risk factors for violence*). If the patient appears to be dangerous, the clinician should consider plans to protect potential victims, such as intensifying therapy if the patient is in outpatient treatment, changing the patient's medication, involving family members to control the patient or to prevent access to weapons, informing the police, hospitalizing the patient, attempting to commit him legally, and warning intended victims after discussing alternatives with the patient.

REFERENCES

Bach-y-Rita, G., et al. "Episodic Dyscontrol: A Study of 130 Violent Patients," *American Journal of Psychiatry* 127:1473-1478, 1971.

Bell, C.C., and Palmer, J.M. "Security Procedures in a Psychiatric Emergency Service," *Journal of the National Medical Association* 73:(9)835-842, September 1981.

Dubin, W.R., and Feld, J.A. "Rapid Tranquilization of the Violent Patient," *American Journal of Emergency Medicine* 7(3):313-320, May 1989.

Dubin, W.R. and Weiss, K.J., "Emergency Psychiatry," in *Psychiatry,* vol. 2. Edited by Michels, R., et al. Philadelphia: J.B. Lippincott Company, 1985.

Dubin, W.R., et al. "Assaults Against Psychiatrists in Outpatient Settings," *Journal of Clinical Psychiatry* 49(9):338-345, September 1988.

Lenefsky, B., et al. "Management of Violent Behaviors," *Perspectives in Psychiatric Care* 16(5/6):212-217, September-December 1978.

Lion, J.R. *Evaluation and Management of the Violent Patient.* Springfield, Ill.: Charles C. Thomas, 1972.

Lion, J.R., et al. "The Self-Referred Violent Patient," *JAMA* 205:91-93, 1968.

Lion, J.R., et al. "Restraining the Violent Patient," *Journal of Psychiatric Nursing and Mental Health Services* 10(2):9-11, March-April 1972.

Monahan, J. "Clinical Prediction of Violent Behavior," *Psychiatric Annals* 12:509-513, 1982.

Salamon, I. "Violent and Aggressive Behavior," in *Psychiatric Emergencies.* Edited by Glick, R.A., et al. New York: Grune & Stratton, 1976.

"Seclusion and Restraint: A Task Force Report #22." Washington, D.C.: American Psychiatric Association, 1985.

Tardiff, K. *Assessment and Management of Violent Patients.* Washington, D.C.: American Psychiatric Press, 1989.

Thackery, M. *Therapeutics for Aggression: Psychological-Physical Crisis Intervention.* New York: Human Sciences Press, 1986.

Van Rybroek, G.J., et al. "Preventive Aggression Devices (PADS): Ambulatory Restraints as an Alternative to Seclusion," *Journal of Clinical Psychiatry* 48(10):401-405, October 1987.

8

SELF-
DESTRUCTIVE
BEHAVIOR

Treating the self-destructive patient is a difficult and often stressful responsibility. The clinician not only must assess the patient's risk of suicide and recommend appropriate therapy but also must confront the underlying question of who is ultimately responsible if the patient commits suicide. Additionally, because of a mistaken belief that all suicide attempts or gestures are purposeful and manipulative, many clinicians have strong negative reactions toward suicidal patients, which further complicates clinical decision making.

Although self-destructive behavior can occur in various settings, emergency department clinicians bear an increased responsibility for self-destructive patients, because the suicide rate in users of psychiatric emergency services is 10 times greater than that in the general population (Hillard, 1983). By following the principles of intervention presented in this chapter, you can ensure that all reasonable treatment options for the suicidal patient have been explored.

▼

IDENTIFYING THE PROBLEM

Self-destructive patients fall into one of three categories: those who have suicidal thoughts but do not try to kill themselves, those who attempt suicide for attention or retaliation but do not intend to kill themselves (suicide gesture), and those who attempt suicide with the intention of fatal consequences. Patients in all diagnostic groups—including those with schizophrenia, depression, mania, and personality disorders—may have suicidal thoughts or make suicide gestures or attempts. In addition, alcohol or drug use can precipitate self-destructive behavior.

Patient safety

Your first priority when presented with a self-destructive patient is to ensure the patient's safety. This can be accomplished by:
• putting the patient in a room free of cords, wires, glass, and other potentially harmful objects
• inspecting the patient's clothes and belongings for weapons or pills
• having a staff or family member remain with the patient
• secluding the patient in a locked, windowless room if he tries to escape
• using soft leather restraints if the patient attempts to inflict self-harm, such as by banging his head
• observing the patient at all times, even in the bathroom
• removing all belts, shoelaces, and stockings from the patient and dressing him in a hospital gown (Hanke, 1984; Dubin and Stolberg, 1981).

Mental status findings

After taking steps to ensure the patient's safety, conduct a mental status examination to determine the patient's suicide risk. A patient is more likely to commit suicide if he exhibits any of the following symptoms:
• *command hallucinations,* which "tell" the patient to act in a self-destructive manner
• *paranoid delusions,* in which the patient feels persecuted or sought after by a known or unknown group of people

• *disorganized thinking,* which prevents the patient from making appropriate treatment choices or cooperating with a treatment plan

• *depressed affect,* in which the patient expresses profound sadness and despondency

• *flat affect,* in which the patient shows no emotion over the suicide thought, gesture, or attempt

• *hopelessness,* in which the patient feels that no alternatives to suicide exist (somatic or nihilistic delusions may contribute to this sense of hopelessness)

• *psychomotor agitation or retardation,* which may indicate the severity of the patient's depression, psychosis, or anxiety

• *disorientation,* which suggests an underlying dementia, delirium, or alcohol or drug intoxication or withdrawal.

A patient's suicidal feelings can range from fleeting ideas to serious intentions. When assessing the patient's thoughts about suicide, do not immediately discuss the self-destructive behavior, especially if the patient appears unprepared to face his suicidal thoughts. Hillard (1983) suggests this gradual line of questioning:

• "Do you feel hopeless?"

• "Do you believe that it isn't worth going on any longer?"

• "Have you thought of hurting yourself?"

• "Have you been concerned that you might lose control and hurt yourself?"

• "Have you planned how you might hurt yourself?"

• "Do you have the means to carry out the plan?"

Physical findings

Your immediate concern when caring for a patient who has attempted suicide should be to assess and treat the patient's physical condition. Obviously, the type of suicide attempt (such as drug overdose, wrist laceration, gunshot wound, or hanging) will dictate the necessary treatment.

When the patient has made a suicide gesture, ensure that the patient has not minimized the problem (for instance, the patient may have swallowed 50 aspirin tablets but state that he took 10). The physical examination also helps determine if the patient has used alcohol or drugs. Assess the patient's heart rate and rhythm, pulse rate, temperature, blood pressure, pupil size, reflexes, gait, and level of consciousness.

Laboratory studies

You will need a laboratory evaluation if you suspect the patient has an underlying medical complication. The type of suicide attempt determines which laboratory studies you should request. An alcohol and drug screen should be part of the diagnostic analysis because the patient may deny or minimize the amount ingested.

Differential diagnosis

The differential diagnosis for self-destructive behavior encompasses all major psychiatric illnesses. These conditions include schizophrenia, major depressive disorder, mania, delirium, alcohol or drug withdrawal or intoxication, dementia, and personality disorders.

▼
INTERPERSONAL INTERVENTION

Interpersonal intervention can be more effective if you keep in mind the possible reasons for suicidal behavior. Underlying motives for self-destructive actions include release from unbearable tension, impulsive response to delusional thinking or command hallucinations, revenge or retaliation toward another person, desire to join a deceased loved one, or religious or political beliefs (Hanke, 1984). Suicide also can be an act of desperation – what appears to be the only solution for a person who feels hopeless or trapped, without a future, alone in the face of overwhelming difficulties.

Evaluating suicide risk

Your primary intervention goal is to determine the risk of suicide. Although no systematic method for assessing ultimate risk has been established, several clinical indicators of high suicide risk have been identified (see *Clinical indicators of high suicide risk*). Remember, however, that these risk factors are not of equal weight; a patient who is psychotic, intoxicated, divorced, widowed, separated, older than age 65, or living alone is at a higher risk for suicide.

When evaluating a patient's suicide risk, consider these factors:

▪ **The seriousness of the suicide attempt.** The more potentially lethal the attempt, the greater the suicide risk. A patient who cuts his wrists or tries to hang or shoot himself has a higher risk for suicide

CLINICAL INDICATORS OF HIGH SUICIDE RISK

The following indicators, if they occur in clusters, suggest an increased risk of suicide:

Epidemiological risk factors
- Separated, divorced, widowed
- Over age 45
- Male
- White
- Recent losses (loved one, health, money, job)
- Protestant
- Spring, fall

Historical data
- Family or personal history of suicidal behavior
- Previous suicide attempts

Concurrent medical conditions
- Chronic or terminal illness
- Chronic pain
- Severe, persistent insomnia
- Hypochondriasis

Concurrent psychopathology
- Poor impulse control
- Poor reality testing
- Psychosis or impaired brain function
- Depression
- Drug or alcohol abuse
- Personality disorders (borderline, paranoid)

Suicidal behavior
- Lethal method and means
- Serious, persistent intent
- Will or serious note written
- High-risk environment (lives alone, has no social supports)

Source: Hanke, 1984, p. 99. Reprinted with permission of the publisher.

than one who takes 10 aspirin tablets. You also must view the seriousness of the attempt in the context of the patient's perceptions. For instance, because aspirin is an over-the-counter drug, a patient may mistakenly believe that taking 50 aspirin tablets is less lethal than taking 10 5-mg diazepam tablets.

■ **The imminence of rescue.** When a patient plans a suicide so that the chance of rescue is remote, the risk for suicide is greater. For example, a person who checks into a hotel and takes an overdose of alcohol and barbiturates at 6:30 p.m. has obviously planned the suicide attempt so that no one will discover him until the next morning. In contrast, someone who takes an overdose of drugs immediately before his spouse arrives home typically has a lower risk for suicide.

■ **The patient's attitude.** The patient's attitude toward the suicide gesture or attempt can indicate future suicide risk. A patient who is glad he survived, one who finds suicidal thoughts and behavior to be unacceptable and frightening, or one who desires help has a lower risk. On the other hand, a patient who is belligerent, stubbornly silent, uncooperative, or indifferent may have a persistent desire for death (Myerson et al., 1976). These negative attitudes can obscure the patient's shame, guilt, and desire to be rescued. Therefore, you should assume that the suicide risk remains sizeable if the patient cannot communicate openly and directly.

A patient who minimizes or denies the risk of death is difficult to assess. The patient may try to convince you that the self-destructive behavior was unintentional. This attitude, common among alcohol and drug abusers, suggests a continued high risk for suicide. Be especially alert when a patient feels reborn after surviving an overdose, coma, or other brush with death. Such a patient may feel elated, claiming that the near-fatal episode has erased his unhappy past. But the patient's elation usually is short-lived—and he again becomes suicidal—when he returns to reality and must face the disappointments of everyday life.

When evaluating a suicidal patient, remain objective, nonjudgmental, and caring. Under no circumstances should you reprimand or belittle the patient, treat the patient with indifference, or minimize the need for intervention. Because a suicidal patient is unusually sensitive to rejection, treat seriously all self-destructive behavior and thoughts, even if you realize early in the interview that the patient did not intend a fatal outcome and was only trying to get attention.

Other staff members also must treat a suicidal patient seriously. The suicidal patient as manipulative and willful creator of his own problems is a common misperception among many staff members, who may resent caring for the patient when "we have really sick patients who need help." They may use the term *suicide gesture* derogatively to characterize the seriousness of the patient's intent, yet many patients who make repeated gestures do eventually kill themselves. Staff members must accept that the suicide gesture or attempt may represent a complete breakdown of the patient's coping mechanisms. Although this behavior appears willful, the patient may be depleted of all psychological resources and incapable of a healthier response. Hostility and rejection by the staff will increase the patient's sense of loneliness and hopelessness, intensifying or prolonging his suicidal impulse.

Crisis intervention

To lower the patient's suicide risk, try to ascertain the reasons for the self-destructive thoughts or behavior and help the patient explore alternative ways to deal with the perceived crisis. Recognize that the suicide attempt or gesture is an active effort by the patient to stop unbearable anguish. Thus, you can defuse the situation by being supportive and caring. If the patient's sense of despair and loneliness can be decreased, he may gain renewed hope of establishing an emotional rapport with others.

To help a highly suicidal person, involve others (supportive relatives, friends, or colleagues), assure the patient that he will be helped, and try to do what the patient wants done (such as referring him to social services for housing, reuniting him with a significant other, or providing relief from symptoms. If that cannot be accomplished, at least move in the direction of the patient's desired goals (Schneidman, 1980).

Be prepared to spend several hours with a self-destructive patient during the initial session. A hurried, harried interview, in which the primary goal is to discharge the patient as quickly as possible, only reaffirms the patient's sense of worthlessness and rejection. A group session that includes the patient, yourself, and other involved staff members is an effective initial intervention. Be sure to introduce all staff members to the patient before the session begins.

Developing a therapeutic relationship

The session should be supportive, with staff members showing empathy. Try to see the world through the patient's eyes. Self-destructive behavior commonly is precipitated by rejection from a lover, spouse, parent, or child. However, the patient's survival suggests ambivalence toward suicide and a desire to live. Instilling hope is the first step in shifting the patient's attitude away from death and toward life.

Offering food and tending to the patient's comfort during the session can help develop a therapeutic alliance. For instance, you might ask the patient, "What can we do for you now?" In answering this question, the patient may divulge the reason for his self-destructive behavior.

When possible, precede interventions by informing the patient, "I'm going to help you now by..." or "The next thing we're going to do for you is...." Using such phrases to announce even routine interventions may help the patient begin to feel accepted, appreciated, and valued. Another helpful intervention is to inquire about and then emphasize the patient's past accomplishments on the job, in a marriage, or during outpatient treatment or hospitalizations. For a patient with repetitive self-destructive behavior, point out that he overcame hopelessness and worthlessness in the past and was able to resume his life. Similarly, if the suicidal behavior results from rejection, note that the patient overcame past rejections and was able to establish other positive relationships.

Explain to the patient that self-destructive behavior is rage directed toward oneself. The patient usually is unaware that he is punishing himself because of anger at someone else. Once the patient understands this, he can begin to develop more constructive ways to channel anger and disappointment.

With the patient's permission, contact family members or friends and request their participation in treatment. Their support and care may enhance the patient's feelings of being wanted and appreciated and ease any feelings of rejection. In addition, family members can provide clinical information that will be helpful in treating the patient. Use discretion when mobilizing such support, however. If relatives or friends are ambivalent or angry, they can exacerbate the patient's feelings of hopelessness and rejection. In such situations, you may choose not to involve them.

SPECIAL PROBLEMS WITH SELF-DESTRUCTIVE PATIENTS

Certain patients create difficulty for the clinician because their behavior prevents the establishment of a therapeutic alliance. Meyerson et al. (1976) describe five types of patients who pose special problems for the clinician.

The depressed patient

The depressed patient feels worthless, guilty, and helpless. If your approach is too kindly and solicitous, the patient's guilt and shame may intensify, preventing the patient from discussing how bad he feels. Thus, the best approach is to conduct yourself as a concerned, albeit neutral, professional. Actively explore the specific details of the patient's self-criticism, anger, and suicidal thoughts and plans, assessing the depth of the patient's depression while trying to appreciate the painfulness of his emotions.

The angry patient

The angry patient may engender further rejection because of immature behavior. You can easily feel trapped in a power struggle with a provocative patient or become angry at the patient for not cooperating. If such a situation goes unchecked, the interview rapidly becomes an extension of the patient's hostile struggle with authority, the angry patient skillfully frustrating your attempts to understand the problem and establish a therapeutic rapport. To overcome these problems, first recognize that your anger at the patient is a response to the patient's displaced anger at another person. Such recognition will allow you to focus on the conflict that prompted the suicide threat. For instance, you might say to the patient, "You must be very angry at someone," which should encourage the patient to discuss the actual target of his anger.

The manipulative patient

The manipulative patient usually tries to prevent you from understanding the situation, perhaps insisting on being hospitalized or not being hospitalized while avoiding any discussion of problems during the interview. An inexperienced clinician may feel compelled to bar the door when such a patient expresses a desire to be in the hospital. This manipulative and demanding behavior, however, provides insight into the patient's way of relating to others and may be a factor in the suicidal crisis. To avoid being manipulated, tell the patient firmly and directly that appropriate treatment decisions cannot be made without sufficient information. The patient may continue to push his demands with such comments as, "Before I can tell you anything, you must promise that...." Instead of giving in to these demands, ask the patient about other situations in which his needs have not been met by others. This approach refocuses the interview on the patient's life and allows discussion of how unsatisfied demands may have led to the patient's suicidal thoughts or behavior.

The patient preoccupied with suicide

A patient may admit to thinking frequently about suicide but deny any intention of carrying out the thought, usually responding with "I think about it, but not really" or "I think about it, but I would never do it. I'm too religious." When interviewing such a patient, ask specific questions that can reveal the patient's intentions, such as whether the patient has made out a will or given away valuables. Conduct a complete mental status examination to assess the patient's suicide risk. A patient who is fully oriented, not psychotic, and without a history of impulsive or suicidal behavior is a low suicide risk (Myerson et al., 1976). Of special concern is the chronically ill, typically elderly patient who wishes "to be allowed to die." Filled with despair, feeling isolated and abandoned, the patient usually is asking the hidden question "Does anyone still care about me?" (Myerson et al, 1976). Although the suicide risk is low in such a patient, you must respond to his concerns in a professional and caring manner.

The patient who telephones

If a patient telephones a hospital or clinic with suicidal threats, ask for the person's name and address and encourage him to come in for an evaluation. A patient who gives truthful information will probably come for help. At serious risk for suicide, however, is the person who refuses an evaluation, especially if he provides evidence of previous self-destructive behavior, has slurred speech, or demonstrates an altered state of consciousness. With such a patient, try to have the call traced by asking a colleague to notify the telephone company on another line, and then inform the police. Although a therapeutic alliance is difficult to establish with such callers, always identify yourself and tell the patient where you can be reached if the call is disconnected. Such information may give the person hope that this is not the last contact he will have.

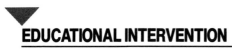

PHARMACOLOGIC INTERVENTION

Psychotic and agitated behavior in a self-destructive patient can be controlled by rapid tranquilization with a neuroleptic medication. Recommended drugs and dosages include haloperidol (Haldol), 10 mg concentrate or 5 mg I.M. every 30 to 60 minutes, or thiothixene (Navane), 20 mg concentrate or 10 mg I.M. every 30 to 60 minutes. For a patient who is not psychotic but extremely anxious and restless, administer 5 to 10 mg of diazepam (Valium) orally or 2 to 4 mg of lorazepam (Ativan) I.M. every 1 to 2 hours. A discharged patient should not be given more than a 1-day supply of medication. Obviously, you must be extremely careful when administering medication to a patient who has attempted suicide with a drug overdose.

EDUCATIONAL INTERVENTION

If you do not address the suicidal patient's hopelessness and depression, the patient will remain at risk for suicide. You can help the patient to understand and cope with depression more successfully by following these guidelines:
• Explain to the patient that depression is a disease, and detail its symptoms.
• Inform the patient that a hallmark of depression is the belief that one will never get well, and point out that this belief is incorrect.
• Explain that depressed patients can get well more quickly with appropriate treatment.
• Emphasize that treatment of depression uses a day-to-day approach (Hillard, 1983).

Other appropriate patient-teaching interventions for the suicidal patient include those listed here:

• Reassure the patient with an adjustment disorder that his feelings and suicidal impulses are transient, and encourage him to seek outpatient evaluation and care.

• Explain the benefits of psychotherapy—facilitating the resolution of the current conflict and developing strategies for preventing future self-destructive behavior.

• Educate a patient whose self-destructive behavior is caused or complicated by alcohol or drugs about the serious medical consequences of substance abuse. In particular, warn the intravenous drug abuser about the risk of acquired immunodeficiency syndrome.

• Provide the substance abuser with information about rehabilitation programs, Alcoholics Anonymous, and other self-help groups.

• Review the prodromal symptoms of psychosis with the patient and family members, and emphasize the need for earlier intervention to prevent or minimize future psychotic episodes.

• Familiarize family members with the state's commitment laws so that they can begin commitment proceedings if the patient refuses treatment.

▼ DISPOSITION

Consider admitting a self-destructive patient to the hospital if *any* of the following criteria apply:

• The patient is psychotic or under the influence of drugs.

• The patient is intoxicated and cannot be treated in the emergency department for 12 or more hours.

• The patient lives alone and no one can stay with him.

• Family and friends can no longer care for the patient in their home.

• The patient's depression and suicidal thoughts persist despite intervention by clinicians, family members, and friends.

• The patient's suicide attempts have increased in frequency or severity.

• You are uncertain of the patient's suicide risk.

Under most circumstances, consider a self-destructive patient ready for discharge if *all* of the following criteria apply:
• The patient's suicide risk is low.
• The patient surrenders the means of committing suicide.
• The crisis that resulted in the suicidal behavior has been resolved.
• The patient's ongoing psychopathology is not severe.
• The patient is oriented and can control his impulses.
• Family members or friends are available for emotional support.
• The patient agrees to participate in a detailed follow-up treatment plan (Hanke, 1984).

If the patient is in ongoing therapy, contact the therapist for a follow-up appointment with the patient the next day. If the patient is not in therapy, arrange for the patient to meet with a therapist within 24 hours, informing the patient of the therapist's name and the time of the appointment. Finally, encourage family members or friends to stay with the patient at all times.

▼
MEDICOLEGAL CONSIDERATIONS

State laws permit involuntary commitment of a person who is demonstrably suicidal, although you should petition for commitment only after the patient refuses voluntary hospitalization. If the patient refuses treatment and cannot be detained legally, contact the patient's family members or friends to alert them to the patient's suicidal behavior.

When treating a self-destructive patient, you can be held liable for professional negligence if you fail to identify the suicide risk, do not try to detain a suicidal person, or prescribe medications that are later used by the patient to attempt suicide. Thorough documentation of the patient's history, examination, and treatment plan are the best protection against charges of negligence.

REFERENCES

Dubin, W.R., and Stolberg, R. *Emergency Psychiatry for the House Officer.* Bridgeport, Conn.: Robert B. Luce, Inc., 1981.

Hanke, N. *Handbook of Emergency Psychiatry.* Lexington, Mass.: Collamore Press, 1984.

Hillard, J.R. "Emergency Management of the Suicidal Patient," in *Psychiatric Emergencies: Intervention and Resolution.* Edited by Walker, J.I. Philadelphia: J.B. Lippincott, 1983.

Myerson, A.T., et al. "Suicide," in *Psychiatric Emergencies.* Edited by Glick, R.A., et al. New York: Grune and Stratton, 1976.

Schneidman, E.S. "Psychotherapy with Suicidal Patients," in *Specialized Techniques in Individual Psychotherapy.* Edited by Karasu, T.B., et al. New York: Brunner/Mazel, 1980.

9

DEPRESSION

A clinician in the psychiatric emergency setting encounters many patients with mild forms of depression, including adjustment disorders and dysthymia. Such patients commonly seek help after suffering a considerable personal, occupational, or financial loss. For example, a patient might feel rejected by a lover, spouse, or parent. For these patients, crisis intervention can significantly alleviate depression and establish a framework for restoring psychological equilibrium.

At the other end of the spectrum are patients enduring major depressive episodes with psychotic features. Patients who are psychotically depressed have severe social impairment and disturbed orientation manifested by delusions, hallucinations, and confusion. Psychotic depression is associated with suicide, repetitive self-destructive acts, and chronic self-neglect.

As with all psychiatric disorders, the clinician must be alert for an underlying medical cause of the patient's depressive symptoms. An organic mood syndrome must be considered part of the differential diagnosis for all depressed patients. Medication, endocrine or neurologic disease, electrolyte imbalance, infection, and substance abuse can also precipitate major depressive episodes, technically called organic mood syndrome.

▼
IDENTIFYING THE PROBLEM

Depression comprises several conditions that differ in clinical presentation, course, pattern of inheritance (some depressive illnesses are genetically inherited), and treatment response (see *Major depressive syndromes* for the features of each depressive disorder). Major depressive episodes usually begin when the patient is in his late 20s but can occur at any age. Symptoms develop over days or weeks. In some cases, however, onset is sudden, especially when depression is related to a psychosocial stressor, such as loss of a job or significant relationship. Duration of the depressive episode varies; untreated episodes can last 6 months or more (*DSM-III-R*, 1987).

Although spontaneous remissions occur in most depressed patients, the risk of suicide and serious medical complications secondary to self-neglect make treatment imperative. About 20% of depressed patients have symptoms that persist for 2 years, and about 15% of these patients commit suicide. Thus, major depression must be considered a life-threatening illness.

Suspect depression in a patient who exhibits the following symptoms (*DSM-III-R*, 1987):

• loss of appetite or significant weight loss or gain (more than 5% of body weight in a month)
• insomnia, characterized by difficulty falling asleep, intermittent sleep during the night, and early waking (1 hour or more earlier than usual)
• hypersomnia, characterized by daytime sleepiness and naps
• sexual disturbance, characterized by loss of interest in intimate sexual relationships
• lack of energy, characterized by complaints of fatigue
• diminished interest in or complete cessation of most activities, including formerly pleasurable ones.

Mental status findings

A depressed patient requires a thorough mental status examination. Significant findings include persistent sadness, psychomotor retardation (ranging from slowed body movement and soft, slurred speech to extreme agitation, pacing, and handwringing), recurring

MAJOR DEPRESSIVE SYNDROMES

Major depressive episode
- Depressed mood
- Diminished pleasure in most or all activities
- Significant weight loss or gain
- Insomnia or hypersomnia daily
- Psychomotor agitation or retardation
- Fatigue or loss of energy
- Feelings of worthlessness
- Inappropriate guilt
- Poor concentration
- Recurrent thoughts of death
- Suicidal ideation, which may be accompanied by hallucinations and delusions

Bipolar disorder, depressed
- All the symptoms of major depressive episode
- History of one or more manic or hypomanic episodes

Dysthymia
(Less severe than major depressive episode)
- Depressed mood most days for at least two years
- In addition, at least two of the following: depressed or overactive appetite, insomnia or hypersomnia, low energy or fatigue, low self-esteem, poor concentration or difficulty making decisions, and feelings of hopelessness

Adjustment disorder with depressed mood
- Reaction to an identifiable psychosocial stressor (or multiple stressors) occurs within 3 months
- Impairment in occupational or school functioning, or in usual social activities and relationships
- Symptoms in excess of a normal and expectable reaction to the stressor
- Maladaptive reaction persists no longer than 6 months, characterized by depressed mood, tearfulness, and feelings of hopelessness

Organic mood syndrome
- Prominent and persistent depressed mood resembling major depressive episode
- Evidence from history, physical examination, or laboratory tests of a specific organic factor judged to be etiologically related to the disturbance
- Not occurring exclusively during the course of delirium

Source: DSM-III-R, 1987. Adapted with permission of the publisher.

thoughts of death and suicide, delusions, cognitive impairment (marked by poor concentration and deficits in recall and short-term memory), worthlessness or guilt (which may be delusional), and hopelessness (difficult to treat because the patient believes that no intervention can eliminate his current problems).

Physical findings
The clinician should conduct a physical and neurologic examination to rule out possible medical causes of depression, including hypokalemia, hyponatremia, Addison's disease, Cushing's syndrome, diabetes, hyperparathyroidism, hyperthyroidism, hypoglycemia, hypothyroidism, encephalitis, drug toxicity, Alzheimer's disease, Huntington's disease, substance abuse, cirrhosis, tuberculosis, hepatitis, and renal failure (Slaby, 1981).

Laboratory studies
A blood chemistry profile, complete blood count, thyroid hormone level, and drug screen are essential. Order further studies based on index of suspicion for the disorders listed above.

Differential diagnosis
If the clinician rules out an organic mood disorder, the focus of the clinical assessment shifts to whether the patient's depression is severe enough to warrant inpatient treatment. If hospitalization is not justified, initial interventions can begin in the emergency setting.

▼
INTERPERSONAL INTERVENTION

Patients who have dysthymia or an adjustment disorder with depressed mood usually arrive in the emergency department (ED) after an upsetting psychosocial stressor. The crisis intervention model of treatment often proves effective in managing nonpsychotic patients with depressive symptoms (Slaby et al., 1981). In a single interview, the clinician can help resolve a conflict by pointing out all options available to the patient. These options can include referral to a housing agency, if that is the patient's primary need, or to other social agencies that can assist the patient with financial, religious, or legal problems. Giving the patient enough time to work through the crisis is vital to the treatment's success. Ideally, other staff members trained in crisis intervention should participate, allowing the patient sufficient time to resolve the crisis without continuous staff involvement.

Acknowledging negative reactions

A clinician sometimes reacts negatively to depressed patients, whose problems may stem from a behavior or life-style not in accord with the clinician's values (for instance, a distraught woman whose relationship with a married man has ended, a man depressed about the breakup of a homosexual relationship, a businessman charged with embezzlement, or a man forbidden to see his children because he is a child abuser). Guard against a superficial, disinterested evaluation or a hostile, angry confrontation. Instead, acknowledge personal feelings of anger, disgust, anxiety, or even attraction and realize that these feelings can impede appropriate evaluation and treatment. If necessary, ask another clinician to speak with the patient.

Conducting the interview

Emergency management of a nonpsychotic patient with depression consists of instilling hope of improvement, clarifying available options, and explaining the benefits of ongoing psychiatric care. Conduct the interview in a quiet room, and pace the discussion so that the patient does not feel hurried. Try to convey warmth, empathy, understanding, and optimism (Tomb, 1988). Enhance the patient's self-esteem by highlighting past accomplishments and strengths. If appropriate, point out that the patient overcame earlier disappointments and adversity. With the patient's permission, contact family members or friends. The intervention is usually more effective when relatives or friends meet with the clinician and patient to plan the patient's next several days. A structured schedule can prevent the patient from dwelling on his problems.

Establishing empathy

The clinician's ability to empathize with the patient can have a substantial impact on the outcome of the intervention (Lane, 1986). Establishing empathy is not easy, though, especially in the ED, where severe illness, disruptive patients, and impending death may intrude. Over time, a clinician may become somewhat hardened to tragedy. To avert such emotional detachment, acknowledge your feelings and perhaps discuss them with colleagues.

An effective way to establish empathy for a patient is to imagine being that patient (Hanke, 1984). The clinician can confirm his understanding of the patient's situation by eliciting feedback from the patient. Feedback can be obtained directly, by asking if the comments about the patient are accurate, or indirectly, by observing nonverbal patient cues, such as good eye contact or nodding yes or no. Further, using key phrases ("It sounds like you..." or "I can see how you...") shows the patient that you are trying to understand his problems, helps gain his trust, gives the patient a chance to confirm or correct your impressions, and puts the patient's experience into words, which may help him understand his feelings.

Maintaining objectivity

Empathy alone is insufficient for an effective intervention. The clinician must also take an objective approach to the patient. Such an approach can provide an alternative explanation of the patient's problem and serve as a guide for data collection and treatment. To illustrate how the clinician can combine empathy with objective observation, Hanke (1984) gives the following example:

A beautiful art student comes into the ED sobbing and distraught. She says, "I'm so ugly, everyone hates me. Ever since my boyfriend left, I sit and cry. When I look in the mirror, I look so old and ugly that I just want to scream." A clinician should respond, "It sounds like you've been feeling pretty bad about yourself since your boyfriend left, but I am a little puzzled how a beautiful young woman like you could see yourself as old and ugly. Do you think you'll always feel this way?"

The first part of the clinician's response indicates participation in the patient's view of herself; the last two comments illustrate the clinician's objective viewpoint. Displaying empathy first is the recommended approach because the patient must feel he is being understood before he will be receptive to an objective viewpoint.

▼
PHARMACOLOGIC INTERVENTION

Interpersonal interventions are much less effective in a patient with severe depression, such as psychotic depression with agitation or depression with severe psychomotor retardation. A severely agitated patient may require rapid tranquilization with high-potency antipsychotic drugs. Recommended doses for acute agitation are thiothixene (Navane) 20 mg oral concentrate or 10 mg I.M., haloperidol (Haldol) 10 mg oral concentrate or 5 mg I.M., or loxapine (Loxitane) 25 mg oral concentrate or 10 mg I.M. In elderly patients, the recommended doses are thiothixene 10 mg concentrate or 5 mg I.M., haloperidol 5 mg concentrate or 2.5 mg I.M., or loxapine 10 mg concentrate or 5 mg I.M. Doses should be given at 30- to 60-minute intervals, and the patient's blood pressure should be taken before each dose is administered.

As a rule, antidepressants should not be given in the ED (Fuchs, 1984). The drugs do not begin to take their desired effect for 10 to 21 days and are associated with adverse side effects that require careful monitoring. Additionally, patients over age 40 (especially those over 65) must have a full medical evaluation before drug treatment is begun. Antidepressants should be limited to an ongoing therapeutic relationship in which adverse effects and clinical response can be observed.

▼
EDUCATIONAL INTERVENTION

Explain to the patient and family the positive prognosis for depression. Tell them that depression responds to psychotherapy and drug treatment, and encourage the patient to seek such additional treatment. Emphasize, however, that discontinuing treatment, even when the patient feels better, may cause a relapse. Teach the family that major depression is a biological illness. Some relatives assume that the patient could become well if he tried harder to overcome symptoms and that lack of effort indicates laziness.

At times, family members may feel emotionally depleted by a patient's long-standing illness. Encourage such members to meet with the treating clinician to express their concerns and feelings.

If the patient is discharged into the care of relatives, refer them to social service resources (such as home nursing or day-care programs) that can assume some of their daily responsibilities to the patient.

Encourage a patient suffering from an adjustment disorder or dysthymia to pursue psychotherapy rather than to rely on drug therapy to resolve distress. A depressed patient may become dependent on a benzodiazepine if the physician tries to alleviate insomnia and anxiety without attempting to change the psychodynamic conflicts that led to the patient's unhappiness.

▼ DISPOSITION

Before discharging a patient, schedule a follow-up appointment, preferably the next day, for further evaluation and treatment. Outpatient therapy for depression should be based not only on the nature and severity of symptoms but also on the patient's psychological makeup and interpersonal style. Crisis intervention, behavior therapy, group and family therapy, and marital counseling are other therapeutic modalities to be considered. A patient requiring medication for anxiety or insomnia should be given a limited quantity of antianxiety drugs, with a prescription not to exceed a 3-day supply. Lorazepam (Ativan) 0.5 to 1 mg twice daily or oxazepam (Serax) 15 to 30 mg twice daily should suffice.

Consider hospitalizing a depressed patient who:

• is at risk for suicide.

• has no family, friends, or other social supports.

• has a long history of depressive illness and does not respond to antidepressant medication as an outpatient.

• experiences command hallucinations.

• cannot independently perform activities of daily living, such as feeding, clothing, and bathing.

• has an associated medical illness that requires treatment.

• requires elevated medication doses.

▼
MEDICOLEGAL CONSIDERATIONS

Patients with depression commonly exhibit self-destructive behavior. Most states allow the clinician to begin civil commitment proceedings for a patient who becomes demonstrably dangerous. In some states, the clinician can commit a patient who cannot perform self-care or whose illness would be life-threatening in a less restrictive environment. Short of commitment, the treatment plan for depression should include safeguards against suicidal behavior, such as voluntary hospitalization or close observation by family members.

Because depressed patients are usually competent to make treatment decisions, the clinician may have to honor a patient's refusal of care. However, a clearly dangerous, psychotic, or demented patient jeopardizes his health by refusing treatment. In such cases, the clinician should work with the family to encourage the patient to accept treatment. Some clinicians apply for civil commitment at this point, thus shifting the burden for making a commitment decision to the judicial system. If the petition is denied, the clinician should make every effort to arrive at a treatment plan that protects the patient. As with all psychiatric emergencies, thoroughly document steps leading to the disposition to avoid future legal complications.

Whether the clinician is liable for the suicide of a depressed patient he discharges depends on the quality of the consultation and supporting documentation. A negligently performed examination – one in which the clinician should have looked for suicidal behavior but failed to do so – provides no sound defense. The clinician should not be liable if a thorough examination has revealed no evidence of suicidal thoughts. Beyond this, the clinician has no duty to control the behavior of patients outside of institutional settings.

▼
SPECIAL SITUATIONS

Most people experience grief after the death of a spouse, parent, child, or other significant person. This response usually runs a benign course, and grieving persons rarely need the attention of a psychiatrist. In some cases, however, grief has a more pathological outcome, and the person requires psychiatric care.

The grieving patient

Grieving is characterized by an intense and repetitive review of one's relationship with the deceased and may be accompanied by depressive symptoms, including fatigue, shortness of breath, dizziness, palpitations, irritability, restlessness, headache, insomnia, appetite loss, inability to organize daily activities, and self-blame. A grieving person may also be preoccupied with the image of the deceased, exhibit hostility toward medical personnel who cared for the deceased, and feel guilty about not having done enough for the deceased. These symptoms usually resolve spontaneously after 3 to 6 months and are part of a healthy response to the loss. Grieving helps the person to lessen attachments to the deceased and regain emotional attachments to others. When a grieving person shows signs of a major depressive episode or displays self-destructive behavior, such as alcohol or drug abuse, psychiatric intervention is necessary.

Initial interventions. The clinician should encourage a grieving patient to review in detail memories of the deceased. Explore the patient's initial reactions to the death and feelings about the deceased. If the patient admits to anger—perhaps because he feels abandoned by the deceased—reassure him that these feelings are normal and will resolve with time. Also, guard against oversedating a grieving patient. Some patients report being so sedated that they do not remember events that occurred immediately before, during, or after the funeral. As a result, they could not adequately express their feelings at the appropriate time.

A patient with a pathological grief reaction becomes withdrawn and isolated. To help such a patient overcome his anguish and maintain social contacts, suggest that he get up and dress every day before noon, schedule household chores and free time for each day, spend time outside the house (running errands, gardening, walking), phone or visit a close friend or relative, and spend a half hour each day writing down feelings about the deceased.

Disposition. If the patient is not psychotic and can be discharged, schedule a follow-up appointment for the next day and, if possible, arrange for the patient to spend time with a family member over the next several days. A patient with extreme anxiety and insomnia may require a benzodiazepine, such as lorazepam 1 mg twice daily. If the patient has symptoms of a nonpsychotic major depressive episode, refer him for continued evaluation and possible treatment with an antidepressant. Some patients with a severe grief reaction may require hospitalization.

Grieving survivors

When a patient dies unexpectedly (such as from a heart attack or automobile accident), the clinician's primary task is to facilitate the survivors' grief (Dubin and Sarnoff, 1986). In most cases, do not inform family members of the death over the telephone but instead tell them that the patient is seriously ill or injured, ask them to come immediately to the hospital, and suggest that a family friend drive them. If a sole survivor is ill or does not have any social support, phone the police department and ask them to contact the survivor. With this approach, a responsible individual is present if the survivor has a catastrophic response to the death.

Initial interventions. Informing relatives of a loved one's death, especially when the patient dies unexpectedly, is one of the clinician's most difficult tasks. Because the physician can answer pertinent medical questions, this task should not be delegated to someone else. Before meeting with the family, prepare to present relevant events in chronological order so that the survivors will have a clear understanding of the circumstances — problems that occurred and actions that were taken. Staff members should be available to meet the family on arrival and escort them to a private area where they can talk with you. Initially, try to determine which survivors will be most stable in the face of devastating news. These persons will be able to make immediate decisions and can later repeat the facts to family members who did not hear or retain what was said. Inform them of the patient's death without using medical jargon or vague descriptions. A gentle but factually informative explanation usually reassures the family that everything reasonable was done to save the patient's life.

Family reactions. The family members' initial response is usually one of numbness, shock, and disbelief. After a few minutes, survivors have various emotional reactions. Some cry easily, while others react with anger, anxiety, guilt, or stoicism. In extreme cases, a survivor may decompensate into psychosis, use defenses such as denial or bewilderment, or have a severe anxiety attack. Encourage family members to express their feelings and to review their final moments with and last memories of the deceased. Refrain from making well-intentioned but ultimately insensitive comments, such as "Everything will be OK" or "It was God's will." Do not immediately offer sedation. Survivors may displace antagonism and anger onto staff members, sometimes accusing hospital staff of being negligent and not doing everything reasonable to save the patient. This anger may represent the survivors' rage at the deceased for abandoning them or their guilt about unresolved conflicts with the deceased. In any event, do not become defensive, guilty, or harried or attempt to counter their anger through rationalization or intellectual explanations. The survivors' anger will ultimately give way to sadness.

Viewing the body. Offer survivors the opportunity to view the body, but don't make them feel guilty if they are reluctant or unwilling to do so. If the body is mutilated, inform family members in advance, and be sure blood and emesis are removed. While the family is viewing the body, remain outside the room, available for support. Survivors should not be hurried. Most family members leave the viewing room within 15 minutes. After family members have viewed the deceased, they may need to sign appropriate papers. At this point, tell them what will happen to the body. If an autopsy is necessary, family members should be told why. Survivors should also be informed of arrangements for transporting the body from the hospital or the medical examiner's office to the funeral home.

Organ donation. The recent increase in organ transport programs imposes a new task on clinicians who deal with survivors of patients who have died suddenly. Such patients may have healthy organs that could benefit a patient waiting for a transplant. Broach the issue of organ donation before family members leave the hospital. For instance, you might ask, "Has your family ever discussed organ or tissue donation?" or "Our hospital offers organ and tissue donation.

Would you like to discuss this further with someone from the transplant program?" If the family expresses an interest, contact the appropriate hospital representative so that discussions can begin immediately. Consider organ donation if the patient meets the general criteria for donor acceptability (those aged 1 day to 65 years who are either brain-dead or on mechanical life-support with intact circulation and who are free from systemic infections, actively transmittable diseases, or cancer).

Concluding the meeting. Conclude the meeting with the patient's survivors by reviewing symptoms of grief and reassuring them that these reactions are normal. Arrange for a family member or friend to stay with a close survivor for the next 24 to 48 hours because suicide is a possibility, especially for a spouse who has been married for many years. Additionally, encourage survivors to discuss the death with their children. An honest discussion can be a positive emotional experience and may help decrease the fantasies and distortions that children can have about death. Adults should not lie, distort the truth, or try to alter the child's feelings about the loss but should express their grief openly; such an approach shows children that an open expression of feelings is acceptable. If the deceased is a parent, young children may require constant reassurance that the surviving parent will not disappear. When adults avoid discussing death with children, they create an atmosphere of apprehension and anxiety, which can be intolerable for children.

REFERENCES

Diagnostic and Statistical Manual of Mental Disorders, 3rd ed., revised. Washington, D.C.: American Psychiatric Association, 1987.

Dubin, W.R., and Sarnoff, J.R. "Sudden Unexpected Death: Intervention with the Survivors," *Annals of Emergency Medicine* 15(1):54-57, January 1986.

Fuchs, R. "Presentation of Depression in the Emergency Setting," in *Emergency Psychiatry: Concepts, Methods, and Practices,* edited by E.L. Bassuck and A.W. Birk. New York: Plenum Press, 1984.

Hanke, N. *Handbook of Emergency Psychiatry.* Lexington, Mass.: Collamore Press, 1984.

Lane, F.E. "Utilizing Physician Empathy with Violent Patients," *American Journal of Psychotherapy* 40(3):448-456, July 1986.

Slaby, A.E. "Emergency Psychiatry: An Update," *Hospital and Community Psychiatry* 32(10):687-698, October 1981.

Slaby, A.E., et al. *Handbook of Psychiatric Emergencies,* 2nd ed. Garden City, N.Y.: Medical Examination Publishing Co., Inc., 1981.

Tomb, D.A. *Psychiatry for the House Officer,* 3rd ed. Baltimore: Williams and Wilkins, 1988.

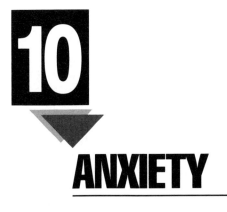

ANXIETY

Fear — a universal response to a perceived threat — prepares one to run away or do battle. At times, this response is maladaptive. Anxiety occurs when mental and physical manifestations of fear develop but serve no purpose, leaving the patient in a state of tension and dread. Because physical symptoms typically accompany anxiety, it is among the most common psychiatric conditions you will see in the emergency setting. This chapter reviews organic anxiety syndrome, panic disorder, generalized anxiety, and anxiety disorders with special symptoms, such as phobias, obsessions, compulsions, and posttraumatic stress disorder.

IDENTIFYING THE PROBLEM: ORGANIC ANXIETY SYNDROME

Anxiety is a mental and physical condition, with major symptoms resulting from stimulation of the autonomic nervous system. The clinician must rule out organic anxiety syndrome before any other anxiety disorder can be diagnosed. In the emergency setting, the differential diagnosis is a routine procedure, although the extent of the examination varies with the clinician's index of suspicion.

Suspect organic anxiety syndrome if the patient has prominent, recurrent panic attacks or generalized anxiety; if the patient's history, physical examination, or laboratory tests indicate a specific organic cause; or if anxiety does not occur exclusively during the course of delirium (*DSM-III-R*, 1987). Organic anxiety syndrome is also likely if the patient is older than age 40 and has no previous psychiatric history, has few psychosocial stressors, abuses alcohol or drugs, or has symptoms that began in response to an illness or medical treatment.

In addition to asking questions about psychosocial stressors and the current illness, focus on the patient's medical history (especially for endocrine disease). Determine if the patient is taking prescribed medication (bronchodilators, stimulants, decongestants, psychotropics, or steroids) or over-the-counter drugs (cold capsules, appetite suppressants, or nasal sprays). Also inquire about the patient's caffeine intake and use of illegal drugs, especially amphetamines, cocaine, and cannabis.

Mental status findings
A patient with organic anxiety syndrome experiences a sense of dread that is not connected to a life event. Some patients begin to avoid situations in which their anxiety could be discovered.

Physical findings
Key findings include mild hypertension and tachycardia, sweating, restlessness, muscle tension, and tremor.

Laboratory studies
Measure any prescription drug blood levels, and obtain blood and urine screens for drugs of abuse, especially cocaine and other stimulants.

Differential diagnosis
The clinician's first task when evaluating an anxious patient is to rule out medical causes of the anxiety (see *Medical disorders associated with anxiety*). Organic anxiety syndrome can also be traced to the patient's use of prescribed medication, including antidepressants, antipsychotics, benzodiazepines, lithium carbonate (Eskalith), aminophylline (Phyllocontin), theophylline (Slo-Phyllin), steroids, sympathomimetics, antiarrhythmics, digoxin (Lanoxin), beta-blockers, reserpine (Serpasil), anabolic steroids, anticholinergics, stimulants, appetite suppressants, isoniazid (Laniazid), nasal decongestants, and salicylates. In some cases, the patient's anxiety

MEDICAL DISORDERS ASSOCIATED WITH ANXIETY

Gastrointestinal system
- Colitis
- Crohn's disease
- Irritable bowel syndrome
- Peptic ulcer disease

Cardiovascular system
- Cardiac arrhythmias
- Cardiomyopathies
- Congestive heart failure
- Coronary insufficiency
- Mitral valve prolapse
- Postmyocardial infarction

Respiratory system
- Asthma
- Chronic obstructive pulmonary disease
- Hyperventilation syndrome
- Pneumothorax
- Pulmonary edema
- Pulmonary embolism

Neurologic system
- Acquired immunodeficiency syndrome
- Dementia and delirium
- Epilepsy
- Essential tremor
- Huntington's disease
- Lupus cerebritis
- Multiple sclerosis
- Parkinson's disease
- Vestibular dysfunction
- Wilson's disease

Endocrine system
- Adrenal insufficiency
- Carcinoid syndrome
- Cushing's syndrome
- Hyperparathyroidism
- Hyperthyroidism
- Hypoglycemia
- Hypothyroidism
- Hypokalemia

may arise from abuse of certain substances, including cannabis (especially high-potency forms), cocaine (especially freebased forms or "crack"), amphetamines, volatile solvents, hallucinogens (especially phencyclidine), sympathomimetic agents, over-the-counter cold remedies, and alcohol.

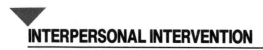

INTERPERSONAL INTERVENTION

Discuss with the patient the nature of his symptoms, and reassure him that they will subside once the underlying medical cause is treated. A psychodynamic or cognitive-behavioral approach is not a component of the interpersonal intervention for a patient with organic anxiety syndrome.

PHARMACOLOGIC INTERVENTION

The clinician should consider pharmacologic intervention for a patient in need of immediate relief from anxiety symptoms or insomnia. However, be cautious when prescribing benzodiazepines for known or suspected drug or alcohol abusers. Substance abusers may enter the emergency department (ED) with complaints of anxiety but have a concealed history of benzodiazepine abuse.

EDUCATIONAL INTERVENTION

If the suspected or known cause of organic anxiety syndrome can be controlled by the patient (for example, by reducing or eliminating caffeine intake), direct educational efforts accordingly. For instance, provide dietary advice or instruct the patient to consult with his primary care physician. Direct compulsive drug users to self-help groups or rehabilitation programs. In addition, because many patients with organic anxiety believe they have a mental disorder, help them to develop a more realistic view of their illness. Tell them that a chemical imbalance has fooled the brain into sensing danger and that this feeling will pass once the imbalance has reversed.

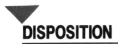

DISPOSITION

Because a medical illness may be causing the patient's anxiety, refer the patient to a primary care physician for further evaluation and treatment rather than to a nonmedical therapist. If the anxiety is caused by drug abuse, firmly recommend that the patient enter a drug detoxification or rehabilitation program.

IDENTIFYING THE PROBLEM: PANIC DISORDER

Panic disorder is a psychiatric illness that can create a subjective sense of emergency for the patient, whose chief complaint may be a "panic attack" or a "heart attack" or feelings of "losing control" or "going crazy." Because serious medical conditions are associated with anxiety and panic disorder, any new patient should receive a thorough physical examination to rule out organic anxiety syndrome (Raj and Sheehan, 1988).

Mental status findings

Mental status findings include depersonalization and a fear of dying or of going crazy. Many patients with panic disorder report an overwhelming need to feel safe and try to avoid places or situations they deem unsafe.

Physical findings

Physical findings include mildly elevated pulse rate and blood pressure; dilated pupils; rapid, shallow breathing; sweating; shortness of breath; chest discomfort; light-headedness; urinary urgency; nausea; diarrhea; and hot flashes or chills. In addition, the patient's history reveals no major psychosocial stressors and no known organic basis for the disorder.

Although most signs and symptoms of panic disorder are physical, medical tests tend to be negative. As a result, an unknowing clinician may dismiss the patient's complaints. Be alert for patients whose chief complaint is a cardiac, gastrointestinal, or neurologic problem, with anxiety as a secondary problem. The clinician can easily misdiagnose the condition, especially if the patient abuses alcohol to escape the anxiety and the clinician fails to recognize the abuse as self-medication (Weiss, 1988).

Laboratory studies

After ruling out myocardial infarction, pulmonary embolism, and other life-threatening conditions, the clinician then orders a drug screen. Organic anxiety syndrome is sometimes caused by drug-induced anxiety and panic states. Treatment for such conditions is obviously different from that for panic disorder alone. Laboratory evaluation should also include blood levels of prescription and nonprescription drugs. For asthmatic patients, serum levels of methylxanthines and sympathomimetic bronchodilators should be measured.

Differential diagnosis

The physical symptoms of panic disorder overlap with several common medical conditions — organic anxiety syndrome, atypical angina or arrhythmia, pulmonary embolism, hypoglycemia, and complex partial epilepsy (Raj and Sheehan, 1988). No standard protocol is followed when evaluating patients with acute anxiety; the clinician is guided by experience and intuition.

The clinician must rule out several other psychiatric conditions when making the differential diagnosis for panic disorder. These conditions include generalized anxiety disorder, adjustment disorder with acute anxiety, post-traumatic stress disorder, major depressive disorder with agitation, somatoform disorders, psychotic disorders, confusional state (typically with dementia), and factitious disorder or compensation neurosis (see *DSM-III-R* for more detailed information on these disorders).

▼

INTERPERSONAL INTERVENTION

Because the clinician does not usually encounter the patient during a panic attack, medication is not the first consideration. And because the panic attack lasts minutes, whereas medications may take a half hour to work, the clinician should not prescribe medication to "catch up" with panic attacks.

Because of the bewildering array of symptoms in panic disorder, the patient needs support in starting treatment. Reassure the patient that he is not "going crazy." Allow him opportunities to express fear and confusion. The patient must understand that panic disorder is a real illness that responds to treatment. Although the patient should be encouraged to enter therapy, help him to realize that much effort will be needed for a successful outcome.

PHARMACOLOGIC INTERVENTION

For a patient who has just had a panic attack and remains fearful and autonomically overaroused, consider prescribing an antianxiety medication. Benzodiazepines are the drugs of choice for such patients. Diazepam (Valium), the best orally absorbed and most rapidly acting benzodiazepine, should be given in oral doses of 5 to 10 mg. Do not administer diazepam I.M., which is a slower route; oral diazepam is effective within 30 minutes.

Although some clinicians routinely prescribe alprazolam (Xanax) as needed for patients with panic disorder, both patient-administered and as-needed doses of alprazolam should be discouraged. The antipanic use of alprazolam requires regular dosing to produce sustained blood levels and must be closely supervised. Alprazolam is usually started at 0.5 mg three times daily. A lasting antipanic effect may require larger doses, prescribed during outpatient treatment.

EDUCATIONAL INTERVENTION

Before discharging the patient, teach him about the illness and its treatment. Explain that although panic disorder is a mental illness, the patient is not "going crazy." Discuss progression of physical and mental symptoms to help the patient understand his behavior (for example, "Given your illness, your behavior is perfectly natural. Now you can do something about it."). The patient should realize that panic disorder does not resolve spontaneously and that he needs treatment, including psychiatric care. Reassure him that medical and psychological treatments can be highly successsful.

In some cases, the patient may suffer from shortness of breath. Because of the resulting hyperventilation, typical symptoms accompanying respiratory alkalosis—air hunger, light-headedness, paresthesias, carpal spasm, or even loss of consciousness—may occur. Education is the most important emergency intervention for hyperventilation. Try to bring its symptoms within the patient's control by having him hyperventilate for a minute or two to replicate the symptoms and then coaching him to slow down the breathing pace or to rebreathe using a bag (the rebreathing maneuver reverses the symptoms of alkalosis). Patients are greatly relieved to learn that symptoms are not part of a life-threatening disorder. Teach the patient to control breathing by mentally counting to 12 before exhaling or by carrying a paper or plastic bag for rebreathing.

DISPOSITION

The patient with panic disorder must understand that ongoing professional care is necessary. Successful therapy entails blocking the attacks, reducing anticipatory anxiety and irrational fears, and dealing with secondary problems (such as interpersonal or occupational difficulties or substance abuse). Therapy may take several months, and the patient must be discouraged from expecting a quick solution. Refer the patient to a psychiatrist skilled in treating panic disorder.

IDENTIFYING THE PROBLEM: GENERALIZED ANXIETY DISORDER

Generalized anxiety disorder (formerly called free-floating anxiety) is characterized by excessive worry and physical symptoms without a perceived stimulus. The illness is usually not a psychiatric emergency, and most patients seek treatment from primary care physicians. A psychiatric emergency can arise, however, if the patient waits until anxiety is unbearable before seeking treatment. Even moderate anxiety can be debilitating and lead to secondary psychosocial, occupational, and medical problems. The varied symptoms of generalized anxiety can occur in any combination. To be diagnosed with generalized anxiety disorder, a patient must have symptoms for 6 months or more.

Mental status findings
Mental status findings include poor concentration, irritability, and edginess.

Physical findings
Physical findings include trembling, twitching, or shakiness; muscle tension, aches, or soreness; restlessness; fatigue; shortness of breath; palpitations or tachycardia; sweating or cold, clammy hands; dry mouth; dizziness or light-headedness; nausea, diarrhea, or other GI distress; hot flashes or chills; frequent urination; difficulty swallowing; exaggerated startle response; and difficulty falling asleep or staying asleep.

Laboratory studies
A drug screen can be helpful in diagnosis and in ruling out benzodiazepine abuse. Otherwise, unless the clinician suspects an underlying medical illness, diagnostic tests are usually left to the patient's primary care physician.

Differential diagnosis
Rule out organic anxiety syndrome (for instance, from cocaine use). Also remember that patients with panic disorder can develop generalized symptoms during their illness.

INTERPERSONAL INTERVENTION

The patient with generalized anxiety disorder develops a set of maladaptive thoughts that correspond to anxious feelings. These thoughts, in turn, perpetuate the anxiety, color the patient's view of the world, and create self-fulfilling failures. For example, the patient may think, "I have no control" or "The world is a dangerous place" or "Everything scares me." To help the patient surmount these problems, the clinician should begin cognitive intervention. McMullin (1986) offers this series of questions to ask the patient in crisis, called brief cognitive restructuring:

- What are you feeling at this moment?
- What triggers your emotions?
- What are you telling yourself right now that is causing you to feel upset?
- What other thoughts cause you to become upset?
- Do you believe that your thoughts are false?
- What evidence do you have that your thoughts are untrue?
- What are your best arguments for disputing these thoughts?
- What practical methods can you use to convince yourself that your thoughts are false?
- If your thoughts are true, what constructive steps can you take to change, avoid, or cope with these thoughts?

PHARMACOLOGIC INTERVENTION

Benzodiazepines are standard drug therapy for anxiety in psychiatric emergency patients. All benzodiazepines are effective sedatives; selection of a particular drug depends on its anticipated onset and duration of action. For instance, diazepam is the most rapidly acting oral agent; lorazepam (Ativan) is most rapidly absorbed intramuscularly and is not associated with paradoxical disinhibition; oxazepam (Serax) produces little euphoria and is rarely abused; and clorazepate (Tranxene) has a very long-acting active metabolite and can be given only once or twice daily. Three of the benzodiazepines — oxazepam, lorazepam, and temazepam (Restoril) — do not require extensive metabolism by liver enzymes, which makes them safer for use in patients with liver disease.

Because parenteral administration of antianxiety drugs is not recommended, prescribe an oral agent. Most patients become calm within 30 to 60 minutes of receiving the medication. Many patients experience a transitory euphoria after taking a benzodiazepine, especially diazepam. Such euphoria can lead to a psychological dependence that interferes with the patient's stopping the drug later in therapy.

Although benzodiazepines are safe and effective, warn the patient about possible adverse effects, including daytime drowsiness, psychomotor impairment (ataxia), cognitive impairment (mental dullness), paradoxical disinhibition, and euphoria leading to abuse.

In addition, the patient may become tolerant to or dependent on the medication, and discontinuing the drug may cause withdrawal symptoms. The clinician must also be aware of possible drug interactions. The combination of a benzodiazepine and ethanol can cause potentiation and disinhibition; a benzodiazepine combined with any depressant drug can cause oversedation, a serious concern because it can lead to falls or automobile accidents.

If the patient with generalized anxiety abuses alcohol or drugs, benzodiazepines may be more of a liability than an asset because of cross-addiction. For such patients, the clinician should prescribe a suitable alternative medication, such as buspirone (BuSpar).

With the exception of buspirone and possibly antihistamines, other psychotropic agents (such as antipsychotics and antidepressants) are not recommended for treatment of generalized anxiety, especially in psychiatric emergency patients. Older agents, such as barbiturates and meprobamate (Equanil), have been replaced by benzodiazepines and should not be prescribed for new patients. Buspirone, a relatively new compound from the chemical class of azapirones, can be used to treat generalized anxiety. This agent is not a benzodiazepine, a sedative, or a controlled substance. Its lack of an immediately perceived effect makes buspirone questionable as an emergency drug. The ideal candidate for buspirone therapy is the patient with long-standing anxiety who does not require as-needed medication and who is willing to delay symptom relief for the week or more required for the drug to take effect. In this way, the patient can avoid the drug's side effects. The dosage of buspirone is 5 mg three times daily for the first week and 10 mg three times daily for the second through fourth weeks. After that, the dosage is increased gradually to 60 mg daily, if needed. Encourage the patient to follow up with outpatient medication supervision, psychotherapy, and other appropriate life-style changes. Buspirone is not the treatment of choice for the patient who needs medication for insomnia or immediate relief from anxiety. Short-term management of insomnia and anxiety can be accomplished with a benzodiazepine or a sedating antihistamine, such as diphenhydramine (Benadryl). Avoid prescribing controlled substances for known or suspected alcohol or drug abusers.

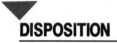

EDUCATIONAL INTERVENTION

The purpose of the emergency visit is not only to relieve anxiety but also to educate and direct the patient toward definitive treatment so that crisis intervention is no longer necessary. Inform the patient that medication, if used, will not be effective on an as-needed basis and that regular dosing with a benzodiazepine or buspirone is required for an anxiety-blocking effect. Encourage the patient to avoid alcohol, caffeine, stimulants, appetite suppressants, tobacco products, and all illicit drugs because these substances can exacerbate anxiety. Because anxiety is accompanied by negative thoughts and other problems in living, suggest psychotherapy, even if the patient is taking medication.

DISPOSITION

Before discharging the patient, reassure him that generalized anxiety disorder is not life-threatening, and refer him to a psychiatrist for follow-up care. Various treatment options include drug therapy with buspirone or a benzodiazepine, psychotherapy, cognitive therapy, and behavior therapy. The clinician need not determine the appropriate therapy at the time of the emergency visit. If the discharge plan includes a prescription for a benzodiazepine, never give the patient more than a 3-day supply. Advise the patient that successful treatment requires an ongoing commitment and regular psychiatric visits — not simply waiting until anxiety is severe enough to make an emergency visit.

IDENTIFYING THE PROBLEM: PHOBIAS, OBSESSIONS, COMPULSIONS, AND P.T.S.D.

Other symptoms that reflect anxiety include phobias (irrational fear and avoidance), obsessions (intrusive, anxiety-producing thoughts), compulsions (repetitive, unwanted behaviors) and post-traumatic stress disorder (PTSD — intrusive reminiscences).

Transient or persistent irrational fear and avoidance is common in adults and normal in children to a degree (Marks, 1987). People with phobias can live comfortably, as long as they avoid the feared object. Phobias are classified as simple, social, and agoraphobia (*DSM-III-R,* 1987). *Simple phobias* include fear of animals (snakes, dogs, insects), blood or injury, dental work, eating (fear of gagging), flying in airplanes, heights, thunderstorms, and enclosed spaces. Common *social phobias* include looking foolish, ridiculous, or ignorant; eating and drinking in public; speaking to persons in authority; blushing, sweating, fainting, or vomiting in front of other people; writing (fear of the hand shaking); and being criticized. *Agoraphobia* is the avoidance pattern associated with panic disorder; that is, avoiding places that the patient associates with a panic attack.

Obsessions and compulsions — unwanted and intrusive thoughts and behaviors — are distressing to the patient and may warrant a visit to the ED. Obsessive thoughts may relate to contaminating others or being contaminated, harming others (for instance, killing an infant), swearing, or being sexually promiscuous. Patients who suffer from compulsions may feel abnormally compelled to clean themselves or objects, repeat words or numbers, check things (especially locks), hoard trash or useless articles, or maintain orderliness by arranging objects. Intensity of symptoms can be so severe that the clinician may suspect a psychosis. Subjectively, the patient feels on the verge of "going crazy" from lack of control over thoughts and deeds. Objectively, the patient may be markedly incapacitated by obsessive thoughts or compulsive acts.

PTSD can develop in victims of traumatic situations — an automobile accident (with or without physical injury), assault and battery, rape, combat, internment in a prisoner-of-war or concentration camp, or severe or protracted illness. Post-traumatic stress symptoms are commonly florid, severe, and disabling. The patient may or may not show immediate distress but will describe an inability to "feel" things (psychic numbing), vivid nightmares, fear of going to sleep, and a startle response to noise. The patient may also experience flashbacks of the traumatic event (which can be dramatic enough to suggest a departure from reality) and may try to avoid reminders of the trauma. During the course of PTSD, which can last for years, the patient may be so disturbed (or family members so disturbed by the patient's behavior) that psychiatric emergency care is needed.

Mental status findings
A phobic patient clearly states his fear; for instance, "You're going to think I'm crazy, but I'm afraid of...." An agoraphobic patient describes symptoms of panic disorder. An obsessive-compulsive patient describes intrusive, unpleasant ideas and irresistible behaviors designed to make the thoughts go away. A patient with PTSD clearly relates symptoms to the original traumatic event.

Physical findings
A patient with compulsive hand washing may show evidence of skin injury. A patient with compulsive hair pulling (trichotillomania) may have spotty baldness.

Laboratory studies
Order appropriate studies if you suspect organic anxiety syndrome.

Differential diagnosis
The primary differential diagnoses are psychosis and organic mental disorders. A patient with schizophrenia may display social avoidance and excessive fearfulness similar to phobic behavior. A psychotic patient may behave idiosyncratically, with auditory hallucinations and strange, ritualistic behavior reminiscent of obsessive-compulsive symptoms. Repetitive and seemingly compulsive behavior is also a characteristic of the chronic amphetamine abuser. Other differential diagnoses include those for phobias (avoidant personality, schizoid or schizotypal personality, schizophrenia, transitory childhood symptoms, normal fear, chronic drug or alcohol abuse, body dysmorphic disorder, and anorexia nervosa), PTSD (dream anxiety and, with accident victims, malingering), and obsessive-compulsive behavior (transitory childhood symptoms, compulsive personality, amphetamine abuse, and culturally sanctioned ritual).

INTERPERSONAL INTERVENTION

To calm the patient, the clinician can use a brief psychotherapy format. Take the patient's complaint seriously, but remind him that his symptoms will not lead to "insanity." Have the patient or a family member carefully recount the history of the problem. This history provides information for a psychosocial formulation, aids in making the differential diagnosis, and allows the patient to express anxious feelings, especially the fear of losing control (Walker, 1983). Anxiety in a phobic patient may or may not be precipitated by an obvious psychosocial stressor. Although phobias may have uncertain causes, reassure the patient that his symptoms can readily respond to behavior therapy.

An obsessive-compulsive patient is difficult to manage, either in an emergency or outpatient setting. Research in obsessive-compulsive disorder suggests that it is a biologically based illness resistant to standard interpersonal intervention. Nevertheless, tell the patient that behavior therapy and pharmacotherapy are promising treatments.

A patient with PTSD can benefit greatly from the opportunity to talk about his experiences, although an open discussion of feelings is not necessarily as healing as time itself. Many PTSD patients feel responsible for their trauma, although few contribute to the problem. Interpreting PTSD as a defense against rage must be done with caution and probably should be left to a psychotherapist, to whom the patient should be referred.

PHARMACOLOGIC INTERVENTION

Use medications sparingly, for several reasons: a definitive treatment is beyond the scope of the emergency setting, the patient should not leave with the impression that drug therapy is a complete treatment, antianxiety medications can block the patient's ability to express feelings, and abuse of and dependence on antianxiety medications can complicate therapy.

The clinician should avoid administering medication to phobic patients, except for those with agoraphobia secondary to panic disorder. A patient with social phobia may request help for a fear of public speaking or flying. For such patients, but not necessarily for those with phobic anxiety in general, a 10- to 20-mg dose of propranolol (Inderal) 1 hour before the feared event will reduce anxiety symptoms. Beta blockers have little long-term usefulness in treating phobia (Gorman, 1989).

A patient with sleep complaints associated with PTSD may require a sedative, such as flurazepam (Dalmane) 15 to 30 mg at bedtime, for no more than 3 days. The definitive drug therapy of PTSD is not established and should not be attempted. Suspect drug abuse in any patient claiming PTSD symptoms who asks for a specific controlled drug (such as diazepam), and alert the patient's prescribing physician. Some PTSD patients enter the ED after taking antipsychotic or antidepressant medication. Before continuing such treatments, attempt to contact the prescribing physician for verification.

The most promising drugs for obsessive-compulsive disorder are antidepressants that block serotonin re-uptake, such as clomipramine (Anafranil) and fluoxetine (Prozac). However, these drugs take several weeks to exert their effect on compulsive behavior and should be used only under the supervision of a psychiatrist involved in the patient's ongoing care, thus ruling out their use in the emergency setting. For an acutely anxious obsessional patient, consider a benzodiazepine, such as lorazepam 1 to 2 mg up to 4 times daily. Some patients respond better to antipsychotic medication, which the clinician should continue cautiously.

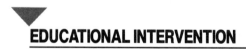

EDUCATIONAL INTERVENTION

Patient teaching entails discussing the therapeutic options available outside the emergency setting, including pharmacotherapy, psychotherapy, and behavior therapy. Additionally, reassure the patient that anxiety does not lead to insanity and that unrealistic fears can be treated without an invasive intervention. Emphasize that phobias, obsessions, and compulsions need not dominate the patient's conscious life, and caution the patient to abstain from alcohol and illegal drugs, which can exacerbate anxiety symptoms.

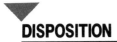

DISPOSITION

Hospitalize a patient who exhibits suicidal ideation or behavior, abuses alcohol or drugs, displays evidence of an underlying psychotic illness, or participates in a medication trial with an experimental agent. Refer all other patients for outpatient treatment. Patients with simple and social phobias respond best to behavior therapy. Refer PTSD patients who are combat veterans to programs run by the Veterans Administration or related groups. Refer rape victims to an appropriate support group, such as Women Against Rape (see Chapter 12). Patients with obsessive-compulsive disorder can benefit from behavior therapy or a program that combines behavioral and pharmacologic approaches. For all patients, stress the need for expert intervention and their active participation in treatment.

MEDICOLEGAL CONSIDERATIONS

Because organic anxiety can mimic common nervousness, a clinician can easily overlook the cause of a patient's complaint. Misdiagnosis or premature discharge can lead to increased morbidity and mortality. To avoid this situation, conduct a thorough examination of all patients.

Never prescribe a benzodiazepine or other controlled drug without determining that the patient needs the drug and will not misuse or abuse it. Document the reason for the prescription in the medical record. Be especially careful not to prematurely discharge a patient given a benzodiazepine because a disinhibition reaction could occur after the patient leaves. All patients who receive benzodiazepines should be observed for at least 2 hours after treatment and should not drive a vehicle for at least 24 hours because of possible psychomotor impairment.

Legal problems can result from errors of commission (prescribing an antidepressant for a suicidal patient, an antipsychotic for a patient with panic disorder, or a benzodiazepine for a drug or alcohol abuser) or omission (failing to detect a serious physical illness, suicidal ideation, or drug withdrawal or toxicity).

The diagnosis of PTSD has been widely used (and probably overused) in the civil courts by plaintiffs' attorneys when attempting to demonstrate psychic injuries after an accident. Sometimes the attorney suggests that the client be examined by a psychiatrist to build a case for PTSD. The clinician may see mild symptoms but not at the level of PTSD. When a patient exaggerates or fabricates post-traumatic symptoms to help the legal case, the clinician must recognize that the patient is malingering, key indicators for which are listed here:

- The patient shows little distress or overacts.
- The referral is made by an attorney, the patient has little to report, and litigation is pending.
- Symptoms present atypically.
- The spouse does not corroborate the symptoms.
- The patient does not cooperate during the examination.
- The patient insists on a diagnosis of PTSD.
- The patient has a history of litigious or antisocial behavior.

If you suspect malingering, consider charting "atypical anxiety" or "impression deferred" rather than allow yourself to be intimidated into a premature diagnosis.

REFERENCES

Diagnostic and Statistical Manual of Mental Disorders, 3rd ed., revised. Washington, D.C.: American Psychiatric Association, 1987.

Gorman, J.M., et al. "A Neuroanatomical Hypothesis for Panic Disorder," *American Journal of Psychiatry* 146(2):148-161, February 1989.

McMullin, R.E. *Handbook of Cognitive Therapy Techniques.* New York: W.W. Norton & Co., 1986.

Marks, I.M. *Fears, Phobias, and Rituals.* New York: Oxford University Press, 1987.

Walker, J.I. *Psychiatric Emergencies: Intervention and Resolution.* Philadelphia: J.B. Lippincott, 1983.

Weiss, K.J. "The Interrelationships Between Anxiety and Alcoholism and Drug Addiction," in *Handbook of Anxiety,* Vol. 2, edited by G. Burrows et al. Amsterdam: Elsevier Science Publishers, 1988.

11

DOMESTIC
ABUSE

Domestic abuse refers to a behavior pattern in which a person repeatedly inflicts physical injury, pain, fear, or mental anguish on another family member. The trauma may be imposed through physical, psychological, sexual, or economic means. Neglect occurs when a caregiver fails to provide basic necessities for a family member.

Many victims of abuse and neglect come to the emergency department (ED) for treatment. Although as many as 21% of all women who use emergency services are battered, only about 1 in 25 is recognized as such by hospital staff and receives care specifically for the abuse (Dickstein, 1988). Similarly, less than 20% of elder abuse incidents come to the attention of authorities (Jones et al., 1988).

Given the frequency of the problem and the difficulty of identifying domestic abuse and neglect, clinicians and staff members should maintain a high index of suspicion. Knowing the signs that suggest domestic violence and neglect can help the clinician determine whether the injury resulted from a pattern of abuse, whether the abused or neglected patient should be separated from the abuser, and whether long-term treatment is necessary.

STAFF REACTIONS TO ABUSE

Treating domestic abuse patients can be stressful for the clinician and other staff members, who typically feel anger toward the abuser. These feelings intensify when the abused patient is helpless, such as a demented elderly patient. Furthermore, when a seemingly competent adult repeatedly returns to the abuser, staff members may become angry with the patient, their anger compounded by futility if they believe they cannot prevent future abuse. Finally, because many abusers have histories of nondomestic violence and threaten to harm anyone who helps the abused, staff members may be fearful of confrontation or of taking action that would anger the abuser.

To reduce their discomfort, some staff members develop myths about domestic abuse. For example, they may view violence as a part of the culture of emergency service patients, who are commonly from poorer socioeconomic groups, or they may come to believe that abused persons provoke violence and purposely choose abusive mates. Anger, fear, and denial are exacerbated if staff members are wrestling with unresolved issues in their own lives. Some staff members may have witnessed violence in their families or may have been victims of child or domestic abuse. Other staff members may provide care to their elderly parents and may feel guilty over a desire to be released from responsibilities, a wish that their parents would die, or anticipation of an inheritance (Lansky, 1985). Consequently, their feelings may influence their response to older abused patients.

Staff members need assistance in handling their feelings toward domestic abuse patients. Supervisors should expect occasionally strong negative reactions from staff members and try to maintain an honest, accepting, and supportive attitude. Realistic concerns of the staff must be separated from myths and distortions. Supervisors can also help staff members by discussing the complex interplay of factors that prevent a simple resolution of the patient's problems. A formal domestic abuse assessment protocol can minimize staff denial that leads to underreporting of abuse (McLeer et al., 1989).

IDENTIFYING THE PROBLEM: SPOUSE ABUSE

The clinician can detect evidence of spouse abuse by thoroughly reviewing the patient's medical history and current symptoms and by carefully assessing the abuser. Inspect and treat the patient's injuries, observe the interaction between the abused and the abuser (if present), and hold separate discussions with each partner.

Assessing the patient

Treating the patient's physical injuries is the first priority. The clinician must then determine whether the injuries were caused by the patient's spouse or partner. Assess conditions surrounding the current episode, including information about threats preceding the abuse and whether economic, physical, verbal, or sexual abuse occurred. During the evaluation, ask the following questions:

• What happened to create these injuries?
• Have you been hurt in the past by your spouse or partner?
• Have you been hurt by other partners?
• Has your spouse or partner hurt others?
• Have you been humiliated by your spouse or partner?
• Has your spouse or partner kept you from using your money?
• Has your spouse or partner threatened you or your family?
• Have you tried to get help? If so, what happened?
• Are you afraid to return home?
• What options do you have?

Obtain a history of the current relationship, including previous types and conditions of abuse. Be especially alert for inconsistencies in the reported cause of the injury. In some cases, the patient's description does not fit the nature of the injury; for example, the patient may attribute a broken bone to a slight shove. In other cases, descriptions taken separately from the patient and other family members are contradictory; for instance, a pregnant woman may claim that she injured her abdomen by falling down the stairs, yet her sister may report that the woman was fighting with her intoxicated boyfriend when she was hurt.

A history of spouse abuse or other domestic abuse in the abused or abuser's family may suggest a current episode of abuse. The abused or abuser may have been abused as a child or witnessed spouse abuse while growing up. Based on these earlier experiences, they may view such behavior as normal. Conditions that increase stress on a family also increase the risk of abuse. Financial difficulties, legal problems, and crowding are common stressors (Dickstein, 1988), as are difficulties with childrearing and changes in family dynamics through birth, illness, marriage, or death.

Mental status findings

According to Dickstein (1988), prolonged abuse can cause symptoms of post-traumatic stress disorder (PTSD). Thus, suspect abuse if the patient exhibits intrusive and fearful thoughts, numbing of normal responsiveness, social withdrawal, diminished interest in normal activities, irritability, and increased startle response (*DSM-III-R,* 1987).

Suicide attempts are also associated with domestic violence (Dickstein, 1988). When questioned, the abused patient may report previous suicide attempts or continual thoughts of suicide or self-harm. Other conditions commonly identified with abuse are depression, anxiety, and panic attacks (Dickstein, 1988; Tilden and Shepherd, 1987). A patient may say, "I've been really depressed lately," or report crying spells, suicidal thoughts, nervousness, dizziness, or palpitations. The patient may also have somatic complaints, such as headache and back pain (McLeer et al., 1989; Tilden and Shepherd, 1987).

Physical findings

Lacerations, contusions, and soft tissue injuries to the head and neck are commonly associated with abuse. Other common injuries include fractures, sprains, burns, intra-abdominal bleeding, and bruises around the wrists or ankles (the result of being physically restrained). You may note signs of a previous injury still healing; for example, an X-ray of a broken arm may reveal evidence of an earlier break.

Assessing the abuser

The clinician usually obtains information about the abuser from the patient because the abuser may not accompany the patient to the ED. Although this information may not be completely accurate, it can be helpful in making clinical decisions about disposition. If the abuser is available for evaluation, the clinician should explore any history of violent behavior.

Abusers usually have diminished impulse control, suggested by a history of head injury or drug or alcohol abuse (Dickstein, 1988). Some psychiatric conditions – psychosis, sociopathy, paranoia, pathological jealousy, mania, and depression – are also associated with poor impulse control. Symptoms of these disorders include delusions (such as extreme, unwarranted jealousy) and auditory or visual hallucinations (for example, thoughts that the abused is "the devil"). Signs of mania include grandiosity, rapid and continuous speech, and decreased need for sleep (*DSM-III-R,* 1987).

Also assess the abuser's attitude. The abuser may not take responsibility for the violent act, may admit committing the violence but feel justified, or may be extremely apologetic in hopes of reuniting with the patient, thus making possible the next incident of abuse. Such attitudes not only reinforce suspicion that abuse has occurred but also provide information about appropriate interventions and help determine whether abuse will continue.

▼
INTERPERSONAL INTERVENTION

Intervention in domestic abuse can be impeded by the abused patient, who may minimize the pain suffered from the attack or claim that the abuser did not really mean any harm. Such acceptance may be accompanied by nonverbal signs of low self-esteem, such as an unkempt appearance and poor eye contact. The patient may also apologize excessively, feel responsible for or deserving of the abuse, or feel unable to live without the abuser, despite the violence. This belief may stem from economic dependence or concerns about separation, especially if previous separations resulted in anxiety, loneliness, or depression. The patient may disguise such concerns with vague rationalizations, typically proclaiming love for the abuser despite believing that the abuser will not change and that abuse will continue.

The abused patient may not want to report the incident or separate from the abuser because of a fear of more serious physical harm. This fear of retaliation may be based on realistic expectations or previous experience. A critical aspect in deciding whether to encourage separation is the risk of continued abuse, which can be determined by evaluating current circumstances (severity of the patient's injury, comorbid conditions in the abused and abuser—especially conditions related to impulse control, family stressors, attitude of the abused, and assessment of the abuser), past history of abuse (circumstances surrounding past episodes, severity of past injuries, frequency of abuse, and attitudes of abused and abuser toward past abuse), and past efforts to stop the abuse (treatment history, involvement with legal authorities, and previous separations). If the risk of further abuse is high, the clinician should encourage a separation.

In determining an appropriate referral placement, the clinician must try to minimize disruption for the family while maintaining adequate protection for the abused patient. The preferred approach is to remove the abuser from the household. Hospital staff may be required to initiate this intervention. To remove the abuser, staff members need to gain the cooperation of the couple, involve other family members to assist in the separation process, and possibly contact legal authorities. Efforts to remove the abuser are not appropriate when he is likely to injure the patient again or is unwilling to cooperate in the separation. Under these circumstances, the clinician should advise the patient to leave home.

ED members should help the patient find a suitable place to stay. Family or friends may be able to provide a temporary residence for the abused patient and any dependents, or the family may already be involved with a social service agency that can assist in residential placement. If no other alternatives exist, the clinician can refer the patient to a shelter. Although the shelter provides protection and ancillary services not available in other settings, moving to one is more disruptive to the family than other options. Staff members should have information about the shelters and their requirements for admission. Critical factors to consider are whether the shelter accepts children, whether its address is anonymous, and whether it offers social services or legal aid.

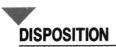

EDUCATIONAL INTERVENTION

Educational interventions are more effective if separation seems unwarranted and the abuser is cooperative. Initially, try to discover the sequence of events that led to the abuse and help the victim and abuser develop strategies to avoid these situations. By reviewing several incidents of abuse with the couple, you can identify key events that typically precede the abuse. For example, the abuse may follow arguments over narrowly defined issues, such as childrearing, money, or drug use. The abuser may hit a wall before striking a partner or spouse or may become violent at specific times during the month, such as just before the next paycheck is received. When the sequence of events is clear, attempt to change the pattern by asking the abused patient to leave before the abuse begins and by asking the abuser to stop using alcohol or illegal drugs. Although the latter suggestion may seem naive, sometimes the shock of recognizing that a loved one has been seriously hurt results in sobriety.

Recognize that the abused patient may have comorbid conditions, such as PTSD, depression, or anxiety disorders. In addition, the abuser may suffer from drug abuse, psychosis, or head trauma. If you suspect any of these conditions exists, refer the patient for treatment. For the patient in acute crisis, empathetic listening and medication may ameliorate symptoms. However, most patients with comorbid disorders require only referral for appropriate treatment. Because motivation to seek help usually increases during a crisis, the abused and the abuser may be more likely to enter a treatment program.

DISPOSITION

Treatment options include private psychotherapists, clinics, and special abuse programs. Self-help and advocacy groups are available for abuse victims and abusers. Participants learn that others have had similar experiences and realize that they are not alone. Support for the couple can also come from extended family, religious organizations, or social agencies.

▼
MEDICOLEGAL CONSIDERATIONS

Become thoroughly familiar with reporting requirements and procedures for initiating legal action. Spouse abuse may constitute assault and battery. Although the victim must bring the charges personally in such cases, the clinician can provide support. For an otherwise physically and mentally fit spouse, the clinician is usually under no legal obligation to notify protective services.

When the abuser is dangerous and unlikely to stay away from the abused, consider involving legal authorities. Arresting the abuser can stop the violence and deter future episodes, especially if the abuser remains in jail. The abuser also learns that his actions have consequences. The courts can enforce a separation through a restraining order. Legal authorities sometimes order the abuser to be evaluated for mental illness or drug abuse and require participation in treatment.

Because legal enforcement of separation varies in different jurisdictions, the clinician and other staff members should know state and local laws regarding spouse abuse, evidence required to arrest and convict the abuser and the likely sentence, and requirements for a restraining order and the consequences if the order is violated.

In some cases, involving the legal system can have negative consequences. The abuser is apt to be angry, which can lead to retaliation – of special concern if the legal system is lenient toward spouse abusers.

▼
IDENTIFYING THE PROBLEM: ELDER ABUSE

Elderly persons can be the victims of passive neglect or physical abuse. The clinician must consider both possibilities when examining an elderly patient. Elder abuse can be difficult to confirm because many victims will not admit to violence or neglect for fear of losing support from the abuser. Sometimes, the elderly victim is too impaired to provide a history of the abuse. As with spouse abuse, the clinician's high index of suspicion is a critical component in making the diagnosis.

The first priority is to treat the physical consequences of the abuse or neglect. Then determine which medications have been prescribed and taken. Contact the patient's primary care physician for information about the medication regimen. Staff members should regulate current doses and examine any physical problems that have resulted from a lack of medication. Refer the patient for treatment of any physical problems that may be contributing to cognitive impairment or emotional instability. These efforts may help reduce the patient's dependency on family members and relieve family stress, thus lessening the risk of further abuse or neglect.

Assessing the patient

The attitude of the abused or neglected elderly patient is comparable to that of the abused spouse. The patient may minimize the problem, appear afraid of the caregiver, or express fears about returning home. When you suspect abuse or neglect, determine the history of such behavior. Ask the patient if he has been hit or otherwise physically harmed in the past or has been deprived of care or necessities. Such questions can reveal a pattern of abuse and allow the patient to report a previous incident, perhaps providing some distance from the current situation and relieving the patient's discomfort about reporting a child or caregiver. Asking about the past also taps the elderly patient's long-term memory, which may be more intact than short-term memory. Also gather information about previous incidents of verbal abuse, threats, restraints, or use of the patient's money without permission.

Mental status findings

Mental status findings in elderly patients who are neglected or abused are the same as those for battered spouses. Withdrawal, depression, anxiety, confusion, suicidal thoughts, low self-esteem, and PTSD are common. The patient may also be disoriented and have an impaired memory.

Physical findings

Physical indicators of elder abuse are similar to those of spouse abuse. Clues to abuse include lacerations, soft tissue injuries, or burns; signs of old injuries at different stages of healing; injuries inconsistent with the explanation given; and delay in seeking medical attention. Signs of sexual abuse, such as evidence of a sexually transmitted disease or pain and bleeding in the genital area, may also be apparent (Bloom et al., 1989).

Signs of neglect differ somewhat from those of abuse. A neglected elderly person may be malnourished or dehydrated and have poor hygiene or pressure sores (Jones et al., 1988; O'Malley et al., 1983). Also be alert for misuse of drugs, including overdosing, underdosing, or inability to obtain medications. Sometimes, you can obtain additional evidence of neglect from the person who brings the elderly patient to the ED; this person may have seen the inside of the patient's home and can comment on the level of cleanliness, the functioning of utilities, and the adequacy of appliances such as walkers or commodes. You may need to speak with this person alone if he is reluctant to speak in front of the patient or other family members.

Assessing the abuser

As with spouse abuse, the abuser may have an impaired impulse control. Impulsivity can result from drug or alcohol use or be a symptom of psychiatric illness. In addition, an elderly abuser may show evidence of dementia. The clinician can assess the specific attitudes of the abuser if he or she is present at the time of the examination. The abuser may be indifferent or angry, fail to assist the patient, show excessive concern about the costs of treatment, or not permit the patient to talk privately with emergency service staff members (Bloom et al., 1989).

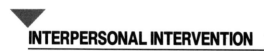

INTERPERSONAL INTERVENTION

Strive to reduce stress on the family by providing support and empathy. Helping the primary caregiver to involve other family members as interim caregivers may provide respite and lower family tension. Further, begin to identify interpersonal conflicts that underlie the abuse. Reactions to the presence of an older relative may vary, depending on the role of the patient and the abuser, the family's life-cycle stage, characteristics of each member, and family circumstances. For example, an adult child may want to care for an elderly parent at home, but the spouse may resent the emotional strains this would entail. Tension increases if the family is already strained by financial worries (such as college expenses) or illness in another member (such as substance abuse). Identifying and clarifying interpersonal conflicts can help determine appropriate referrals and may motivate the family to seek treatment.

Caring for a patient with Alzheimer's disease or another senile dementia is particularly difficult. As the disease progresses, the patient's impulse control and judgment deteriorate, and he cannot manage even the most basic activities of daily living. As a result, the caregiver must provide constant supervision for someone who becomes increasingly agitated, paranoid, and demanding. Not surprisingly, several characteristics of Alzheimer's disease – including dependency, cognitive impairment, and provocative behavior – are associated with elder abuse (Kosberg, 1988). Mounting stress may eventually overwhelm the caregiver, who may react by withholding care or by restraining or striking the patient (Yatzkan, 1988; O'Malley et al., 1983).

EDUCATIONAL INTERVENTION

Although usually initiated in the emergency setting, treatment for the patient, the abuser, and other family members must continue outside the hospital. Thus, the clinician and other staff should inform the family of appropriate community resources (such as individual counseling or family therapy) and make necessary referrals. These resources can provide emotional support, treatment of comorbid conditions (such as substance abuse, psychosis, depression, or dementia), and counseling to improve family communication and resolve interpersonal conflicts.

Other community resources, such as support groups for caregivers of Alzheimer's patients, offer family members the opportunity to share information and personal experiences. Visiting nurse or homemaker services, day programs, and senior citizen centers meet the needs of elderly persons at various levels of functioning and provide a social outlet to minimize isolation. These programs can reduce family tensions by providing care and attention to the patient and a much-needed respite for caregivers. Welfare or family service agencies can provide additional social support and financial assistance in coping with economic hardship or overcrowded living conditions, either of which may contribute to violent behavior.

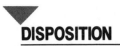

DISPOSITION

As with spouse abuse, if the risk of severe or permanent injury to an elderly patient is high, consider separating the patient from the abuser. Evaluate the family's stress level and interpersonal conflicts, severity of the patient's current injuries, and the abuser's past patterns of violence. Consider several alternative placements, although some are available only on a short-term basis. Relatives or friends may be able to provide care, sometimes for extended periods. Shelters offer another alternative, but the need to treat medical problems related to the abuse or neglect may preclude such a referral. Nursing home placement is another option. In some circumstances, the clinician may need to hospitalize the abused patient for medical management and protection.

MEDICOLEGAL CONSIDERATIONS

Some states require clinicians (and other citizens) to report suspected or known cases of elder abuse or abuse of persons in boarding homes or institutions. Failure to report abuse can lead to criminal or civil penalties. The clinician should become familiar with the protocol for reporting such abuse and thoroughly document evidence of the abuse.

REFERENCES

Bloom, J.S., et al. "Detecting Elder Abuse: A Guide for Physicians," *Geriatrics* 44(6):40-44, June 1989.

Diagnostic and Statistical Manual of Mental Disorders, 3rd ed., revised. Washington, D.C.: American Psychiatric Association, 1987.

Dickstein, L.J. "Spouse Abuse and Other Domestic Violence," *Psychiatric Clinics of North America* 11(4):611-628, December 1988.

Jones, J., et al. "Emergency Department Protocol for the Diagnosis and Evaluation of Geriatric Abuse," *Annals of Emergency Medicine* 17(10):1006-1015, October 1988.

Kosberg, J. "Preventing Elder Abuse: Identification of High Risk Factors Prior to Placement Decisions," *The Gerontologist* 28:43-50, 1988.

Lansky, M.R. "Family Psychotherapy of the Patient with Chronic Organic Brain Syndrome," in *Family Approaches to Major Psychiatric Disorders,* edited by M.R. Lansky. Washington, D.C.: American Psychiatric Association, 1985.

McLeer, S.V., et al. "Education Is Not Enough: A System's Failure in Protecting Battered Women," *Annals of Emergency Medicine* 18(6):651-653, June 1989.

O'Malley, T.A., et al. "Identifying and Preventing Family-Mediated Abuse and Neglect of Elderly Persons," *Annals of Internal Medicine* 98(6):998-1005, June 1983.

Tilden, V.P., and Sheperd, P.H. "Increasing the Rate of Identification of Battered Women in an Emergency Department: Use of a Nursing Protocol," *Research in Nursing and Health* 10(4):209-215, August 1987.

Yatzkan, E.S. "Emergency Situations for Patients and Caregivers," in *Understanding Alzheimer's Disease,* edited by M.K. Aronson. New York: Charles Scribner's Sons, 1988.

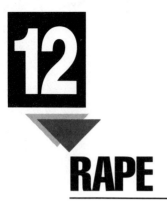

RAPE

Rape is a violent crime, most often perpetrated by men against women. Largely because of the women's movement, popular misconceptions and attitudes toward rape and rape victims have been slowly changing. In addition, crisis intervention centers have developed better support systems and more sophisticated evaluation techniques to help victims of sexual assault.

To receive help at most rape intervention centers, a victim must report the assault to many people – police detectives, physicians, nurses, rape counselors – in addition to her immediate social circle of husband or lover, children, parents, and friends. Thus, the clinician must offer professional services with compassion and respect for the patient and remember that rape is ultimately an intensely personal crisis.

Although the long-term effects of rape need further study, insight-oriented psychotherapy can be a vital part of long-term recovery (Rose, 1986). This chapter reviews the various aspects of emergency care of the rape victim and discusses supportive psychological interventions.

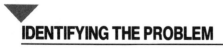

IDENTIFYING THE PROBLEM

When the patient's chief complaint is sexual assault, obtain a history of the event through direct but sensitive questioning, but allow the woman to talk spontaneously about what happened. The patient may have either acute or delayed symptoms, depending on when the attack occurred. To provide adequate physical care, you will have to inquire about particular details of the attack (such as oral or anal penetration) if the victim does not provide them. Alternate between open- and close-ended questions. For example, if a woman enters the emergency service and says, "I was raped today. I feel like I'm going to die," your first question should be open-ended: "Can you tell me what happened, from beginning to end?" When events are not clear, ask close-ended questions: "Were you threatened with a weapon?" or "Were you forced to perform oral sex on the attacker?" Remain calm and empathetic when asking these questions. When the chief complaint includes suicidal thoughts, ask direct questions: "Are you thinking about ending your life right now?" or "Have you tried to kill yourself since this attack occurred?"

Occasionally, the history and mental status examination of a patient who complains of sexual assault clearly point to an acutely manic or paranoid psychosis. The history may be unreliable and erratic because of the patient's thought disorder. In these cases, treat the psychosis first and complete the routine protocol for rape victims when the patient is more coherent. Patients who are acutely psychotic and disorganized may be at higher risk for becoming victims of rape and other violent crimes. Between 70% and 80% of psychiatric inpatients have been victims of physical or sexual assault (Jacobson and Richardson, 1987). These patients may quickly incorporate the actual traumatic event into a paranoid delusional system (for example, ideas of persecution).

The patient may consciously conceal or unconsciously repress sexual trauma. Although a patient may come to a crisis center or outpatient psychotherapy session with symptoms of delayed post-traumatic stress disorder, she does not spontaneously reveal that she has been raped. Several cases of self-cutting have been reported as the primary symptom after rape (Greenspan and Samuel, 1989). As a result, you should routinely include sensitive questioning about the possibility of sexual assault as part of any emergency psychiatric interview. And because the rape victim may be a drug or alcohol abuser, you should ask all patients about substance abuse and order drug screens if appropriate.

Mental status findings

Concentration and judgment may be somewhat impaired secondary to the victim's shock. Suicidal ideation, gestures, or attempts are more likely than homicidal or aggressive acts. Dissociative states may develop later. Prominent findings in the delayed stage include disorientation, confusion, derealization (severe feeling of detachment), and depersonalization.

Rape trauma syndrome, a variant of post-traumatic stress disorder, has acute and delayed stages. The acute stage begins within 24 hours of the assault and may last for several weeks. Although rape victims may seek help during the acute stage, many victims report the attack weeks or months later. Psychological symptoms can range from numbness, disbelief, panic, severe anxiety, anger, self-blame, humiliation, and depression to outer calmness, compliance, glibness, and talkativeness.

The delayed stage usually begins several weeks after the assault and can persist for months or years. Symptoms include anxiety, nightmares, flashbacks, guilt, depression, anger, disinterest in sex, anorgasmia, and suicidal ideation. The intensity and duration of symptoms vary greatly among patients. Much depends on the woman's coping skills, social supports, and preassault level of functioning. Because the details and nature of the assault are of great importance, assess the extent of violence, the type of sexual attack, the number of attackers, and the availability of safety after the assault. This information can help you anticipate post-traumatic symptoms.

Many victims are threatened with another attack or with death if they report the rape. In these situations, continued reminders of the traumatic assault in the victim's everyday life complicate recovery.

Physical findings

Conduct a comprehensive and detailed physical examination of the victim, documenting locations and dimensions of all injuries—bruises, fractures, lacerations, scratches, and inflammation of soft tissue and mucosae. All rape victims must have a pelvic examination. A female nurse should stay in the room with the patient during the examination, especially if the examiner is male. As much as possible, avoid what has been called a "second rape" of the victim—potentially invasive and subjectively threatening aspects of the emergency department (ED) examination. (See *Protocol for examining a rape victim,* pages 190 and 191, for more detailed information on the examination.)

Laboratory studies

Appropriate laboratory tests are discussed in *Protocol for examining a rape victim,* pages 190 and 191.

Differential diagnosis

The differential diagnosis for rape is not complex. Most rape victims enter the ED with a clearly stated chief complaint, which leaves few other diagnoses to rule out. Alternative diagnoses are delusional disorder (as part of schizophrenia, bipolar affective disorder, or a toxic psychosis) and dissociative disorder. Concurrent diagnoses of alcohol or substance abuse can occur.

▼
INTERPERSONAL INTERVENTION

The clinician should be supportive but not intrusive with the patient who has just been raped and should view the interaction with the rape victim as psychotherapeutic, from gathering the history to arranging follow-up care. When possible, interview the rape victim in a safe and quiet place. Recovery from the assault begins almost immediately. Facilitating and supporting this recovery is the responsibility of the physicians, nurses, and counselors in the ED.

Staff members should not pass judgment on a patient who reports a rape. A disapproving or negative attitude directly affects the victim's level of comfort in discussing the rape. More important, a judgmental or uncaring attitude may block the woman's natural expression of emotions or intensify her feelings of self-blame, guilt, and helplessness.

Familiarity with the typical range of responses to trauma can facilitate interpersonal interventions. For example, the question "Do you blame yourself for this attack?" can lead to a discussion of the patient's guilt and shame. Keep in mind that issues addressed in the first encounter cannot be resolved immediately, but discussing the problems openly sets the stage for continued work and offers the woman hope of gaining control over her reactions to the trau-

PROTOCOL FOR EXAMINING A RAPE VICTIM

Most crisis centers have a medical protocol for clinicians who examine rape victims. This protocol outlines the details of the examination for medicolegal purposes, along with appropriate tests and treatments for sexually transmitted diseases and pregnancy. Whether victims should be screened for human immunodeficiency virus is debatable; the value of immediate testing has not been established. The standard protocol of Thomas Jefferson University Hospital in Philadelphia is presented here:

• A gynecologist (6 p.m. to midnight, 7 days a week) or the emergency medicine resident (all other times) should respond when a rape victim age 14 years or older arrives in the emergency department (ED). A pediatrician (8 a.m. to 5 p.m., Monday through Friday) or the emergency medicine resident (all other times) should respond for children younger than age 14. The emergency medicine resident should examine male rape victims age 14 or older. Consider hospitalizing a child if she would be placed in jeopardy by returning home. Sexual assault is a form of child abuse.

• A registered nurse must be present during the examination and treatment to serve as a witness (preferably the support person, to maintain continuity). Police officers should not be present during the examination and treatment.

• Obtain a gynecological history if appropriate. Document the physical examination on the history and sexual assault form and the ED form. Record pertinent medical history (last menstrual period, contraceptive use, presence of venereal disease) on the ED form.

• Perform a general examination, documenting the patient's general physical appearance and demeanor, marks on her body or clothing, bleeding, and physical trauma. Record any physical trauma reported by the victim and any symptoms of emotional trauma.

• Perform a vaginal examination, which is essential to determine injury. Use a nonlubricated, water-moistened speculum (a small speculum for a victim whose tissues are especially sensitive). Inspect the vulva for evidence of trauma and the cervix and vaginal walls for lacerations, contusions, or abrasions. Obtain appropriate specimens. Then perform a bimanual examination to determine the size of the uterus and ovaries. Note that a speculum examination may not always be necessary or appropriate. The examiner may choose to collect specimens with swabs or saline washes. For male victims, complete a full genital and anal examination.

• Order appropriate laboratory tests, which can detect untoward consequences of sexual contact (sexually transmitted diseases, pregnancy) and provide evidence for possible assault charges. Using the department's rape kit, collect necessary specimens, which will be processed by the police crime laboratory. If the crime occurred in the last 7 days, relevant specimens include a blood sample; saliva sample; two swabs from the areas of alleged penetration (vagina, rectum, mouth), placed in a red-top

---

PROTOCOL FOR EXAMINING A RAPE VICTIM *(continued)*

tube; hair samples when they are obviously out of place (pubic hair forced into the vagina, hair in the pubic area of children, hair a different color from that of the patient); any extraneous fibers or particles (paint, wood, blood, semen), which should be placed on a sheet of clean paper, folded to hold the sample, put in an envelope, and sealed; and the victim's clothing, especially undergarments, if soiled, torn, or containing material that could be used as evidence. Seal all evidence with tape and keep it in the refrigerator until delivered to the police. Always test the patient for venereal disease regardless of when the assault occurred. Draw a blood sample for a rapid plasma reagin test, and obtain cultures from the cervical canal, throat, or rectum, as appropriate. Pregnancy testing can be done at the examiner's discretion.

• Treat all life-threatening injuries first. All victims should receive preventive therapy against urethral, cervical, anal, and oral gonorrhea: 125 mg I.M. of ceftriaxone (Rocephin) in patients who weigh less than 100 lb (45 kg) and 250 mg I.M. for those who weigh 100 lb or more. If the patient is allergic to penicillin, 40 mg/kg of spectinomycin (Trobicin) I.M. (maximum dose, 2 g) should be given in a single dose. Both drugs must be followed by either 500 mg of tetracycline (Bristacycline) four times daily for 7 days or 100 mg of doxycycline (Vibramicin) twice daily for 7 days (adults only). Although pediatric victims can be treated prophylactically with either ceftriaxone or spectinomycin, the clinician should wait for positive culture results before initiating drug therapy.

Source: Zeccardi, 1988. Adapted courtesy of Thomas Jefferson University Hospital.

---

matic event. Avoid exploring areas that are neither relevant nor helpful to the woman. Questioning a rape victim about sexual fantasies or gathering a complete history of sexual partners is inappropriate during the initial interview. These issues can be covered later in the patient's recovery, if appropriate.

If the rape victim is female and the perpetrator male, a female counselor should conduct the interview, if possible. In most EDs, a female nurse is present even when the examining physician is a woman, since the pelvic examination is potentially distressing. If the rape victim expresses a preference for a female physician, her request should be respected, if possible.

Most rape victims identify at least one person—husband, lover, parent, or friend—to whom they can turn for social support. The counselor should offer significant support to this person, especially by providing information about rape trauma syndrome. However, maintain confidentiality about the specifics of the sexual assault, and release no details without the patient's consent.

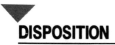

PHARMACOLOGIC INTERVENTION

Before administering any medication to a rape victim, the clinician must obtain her informed consent. Minor tranquilizers are the most commonly used pharmacologic agents in the psychiatric emergency treatment of sexual assault. Psychotropic medications are rarely used. The primary indication for a minor tranquilizer is severe anxiety or panic that does not respond to supportive psychological intervention. Recommended doses are alprazolam (Xanax) 0.25 to 0.5 mg by mouth or lorazepam (Ativan) 1 to 2 mg by mouth. One dose is usually enough to make the patient feel calmer and more in control. When the patient has an underlying diagnosis of schizophrenia, bipolar affective illness, or another psychotic disorder, the clinician may need to administer a dose of the patient's standard neuroleptic medication. Neuroleptic agents should be given if the patient is agitated or hallucinating or has disorganized thoughts.

EDUCATIONAL INTERVENTION

Educate the patient about the typical emotional responses to trauma (see "Mental status findings" above). Because a sense of isolation commonly accompanies the rape victim's panic and shock, learning that others have undergone the same experience can be reassuring. This premise is the basis for the follow-up support groups offered by many rape counseling centers.

DISPOSITION

Most rape victims can be allowed to return home after examination and treatment. Try to ensure that the patient has a supportive person at home, and refer the woman to an appropriate follow-up agency (medical clinic, rape counseling center, or psychiatric service).

MEDICOLEGAL CONSIDERATIONS

Laws regarding notification of authorities vary from state to state. Most rape intervention centers have written protocols that detail these requirements. Clinicians and other staff members are obligated to notify the police of any injury that occurred as the result of a crime. In cases involving children, the clinician must make a full report to the child welfare division of the state government. A telephone hotline is usually available for this purpose.

Medical information about the sexual assault can be released only with the written consent of the patient or by a subpoena or court order. When recording the history, do not describe the events with the assumption that a rape has or has not taken place. Always refer to the sexual assault as "alleged," and clearly indicate descriptions or direct quotations from the patient as such. Medical personnel do not determine whether a crime has occurred; that determination is left to the judicial system.

The clinician and the crisis counselor are responsible for accurately describing their findings. When no one has witnessed the rape, the clinician's observations and recognition of trauma are the only corroborating evidence for a criminal investigation and trial. Careful notation of all signs of physical and sexual assault must be made in the medical record. The likelihood of medical personnel being subpoenaed by the court is lessened if medical documentation is thorough and complete.

REFERENCES

Greenspan, G., and Samuel, S. "Self-Cutting after Rape," *American Journal of Psychiatry* 146(6):789-790, June 1989.

Jacobson, A., and Richardson, B. "Assault Experiences of 100 Psychiatric Inpatients: Evidence of the Need for Routine Inquiry," *American Journal of Psychiatry* 144(7):908-913, July 1987.

Rose, D. "Worse than Death: Psychodynamics of Rape Victims and the Need for Psychotherapy," *American Journal of Psychiatry* 143(7):817-824, July 1986.

Zeccardi, J. "Rape Victim Protocol." Philadelphia: Thomas Jefferson University Hospital, 1988 (unpublished).

13

CHILD AND
ADOLESCENT
EMERGENCIES

Psychiatric emergencies in children and adolescents can be similar to or different from those in adults. For instance, suicide, violent behavior, and drug and alcohol abuse are seen in persons of all ages, whereas runaway behavior is unique to children and adolescents because they are physically, emotionally, and legally dependent on a parent or adult guardian.

When evaluating the child in the emergency service, the clinician must ensure the child's physical safety, assess and intervene with the parent or caregiver, and adhere to any legal requirements applicable to minors. A complete emergency psychiatric evaluation includes the chief complaint, the present illness and precipitating stress, the family history and composition, the child's developmental and medical history as relevant, a detailed interview with the child and family, and a mental status examination of the child (Robinson, 1986).

This chapter reviews suicidal, violent, abusive, and addictive behavioral emergencies in children and adolescents and outlines specific treatment considerations for these problems.

IDENTIFYING THE PROBLEM: SUICIDAL BEHAVIOR

Suicidal behavior is the most common psychiatric emergency in children and adolescents. Suicide is the third most common cause of death in this age-group, and the suicide rate among children and adolescents is rapidly increasing. Girls contemplate suicide three times more frequently than boys, yet boys kill themselves almost three times more often than girls (Khan, 1979; Pfeffer, 1981).

The clinician must take seriously any suicidal behavior, regardless of the patient's age. Although younger children may not understand the finality of death, their consideration of death as a solution to an unbearable situation is as dangerous as an older child planning a suicide, and the clinician must help the patient realize that alternatives to suicide exist. Suicidal behavior can be acute or chronic, intentional or unintentional, planned or impulsive, and more or less ambivalently executed.

The suicidal child or adolescent is usually brought to the emergency department (ED) by a parent, guardian, relative, friend, school nurse or counselor, or religious advisor, and the accompanying person may describe the chief complaint (accident, overdose, or self-mutilation). Only after the clinician inquires about the details of the event does the patient usually admit to having suicidal thoughts, wishes, or plans or to being angry or depressed. Even more investigation is needed for the patient to reveal a relationship between external events or stressors and the feelings, thoughts, and actions that resulted in the psychiatric emergency.

The patient who is admitted with a serious injury or overdose should be medically treated first, then referred for psychiatric evaluation only when out of immediate danger. Depending on the severity of the medical condition, the patient may not be able to speak about the event for hours or days. In all cases, assess the probability of future suicidal behavior and have a skilled staff available if the patient tries to harm himself while receiving medical care. Medical management and psychiatric evaluation can occur simultaneously if the patient is conscious and cooperative. If the patient does not cooperate, use any means necessary, including restraints, to prevent further self-destructive behavior.

To assess the patient's motivation and likelihood of immediate suicidal risk, establish a relationship with the patient and his parents. Speak with the child first, then the parents, and then the family together, if possible. Parents can provide information about family stressors, previous suicidal gestures or attempts, and family history of suicidal behavior. In this way, you can construct a complete picture of the situation and discuss the urgency of intervention with the patient and the parents.

To determine the risk of future suicidal behavior, document all indicators of high suicide risk. Future suicide attempts are more likely if the patient:
• has poor family support or is living away from home.
• has a family history of suicide attempts, depression, or drug or alcohol abuse.
• has a concomitant psychiatric diagnosis.
• expresses a wish to die.
• has attempted suicide.
• feels depressed, helpless, hopeless, and worthless.
• cannot establish a satisfactory relationship with the clinician.

Mental status findings
Determine whether the patient is aware of the seriousness of his behavior and the finality of death, whether the patient is experiencing command hallucinations that order suicidal behavior, and whether the patient exhibits signs of a psychosis (bizarre thoughts, delusions, loose associations, and other noncommand hallucinations). For the mental status examination, evaluate the patient's impulse control (ability to control anger, anxiety, or other powerful emotions that may result in dangerous behavior) and mood and affect (feelings of anger, depression, fear, guilt, hopelessness, helplessness, or worthlessness). Document signs of drug or alcohol intoxication or withdrawal—slurred and incoherent speech, disorientation, memory deficits, and lowered or heightened level of consciousness.

Physical findings
Note any abnormalities that may pertain to the suicidal behavior. For example, depression may be caused by an underlying medical illness, such as chronic infection, endocrine disorders (hypothy-

roidism, hyperparathyroidism, Addison's disease, diabetes mellitus), neoplasia, intoxication (from alcohol, sedatives, marijuana, stimulants), or withdrawal (from stimulants, especially cocaine). Physical findings can also indicate an underlying illness or handicap that causes the patient to feel hopeless, ashamed, or frightened enough to contemplate and carry out suicide. For instance, patients who are blind, deaf, or mentally impaired and those with learning disabilities (such as dyslexia) or a condition that requires frequent or regular medication (insulin-dependent diabetes) are more likely to become depressed. Because children, especially adolescents, respond to peer pressure and because adolescents are preoccupied with their body shape, size, and function, any physical handicap can have a profound impact. Fear of rejection by the peer group may trigger depression and suicidal behavior.

Family assessment

Suicidal behavior in a child or adolescent is a family problem. The clinician must assess the parents' role in the behavior as well as their response to it and their ability and willingness to safeguard the child. Suicidal behavior in a nonpsychotic patient represents the patient's maladaptive attempt to rectify a breakdown in child-parent communication. Such behavior demands a prompt, nonjudgmental, and caring response from the parents. Whether the parents can respond in this manner depends on how the family as a whole behaves in the crisis.

Differential diagnosis

The most important differential diagnosis is "accidental" behavior. Some psychiatrists believe that most serious accidents are the result of unconscious suicidal or homicidal impulses. The patient's emotional response to an accident may be the first and only clue to more serious ramifications. Even with very young children who accidentally ingest poisons, a certain amount of parental negligence may be present.

The clinician must also differentiate between a suicidal gesture (parasuicide) and an attempt. To make this clinical judgment, consider that a gesture is typically less serious than an attempt and more likely a planned effort to manipulate another person rather than an attempt to die; that a person making a suicide gesture is more ambivalent about living and dying and more likely to want help; that a gesture is more likely to represent a plea for help; and that persons may make repeated gestures, which can ultimately result in their death.

▼ INTERPERSONAL INTERVENTION

Intervention and treatment start with the initial evaluation and are primarily interpersonal and family-based. Begin to establish a rapport with the child by speaking his language, paying attention to the direction he takes during the interview, attending to objects or toys he brings to the hospital, maintaining a nonjudgmental attitude, and allowing enough time to listen to him.

To assess the severity of the situation, ask direct questions about the patient's behavior; that is, whether the attempt was planned or impulsive, whether the patient was alone, whether the patient requested help for a problem, and whether the patient left a note. Also consider the seriousness of the injury, even when the patient reports no earnest intent to commit suicide or claims accidental ingestion. Adolescents and children do commit suicide by accident: they may misjudge the depth of a cut, the placement of a gun, the number of pills to take, or the potential response of another person.

Obtain as many details as possible about the suicide attempt to evaluate the patient's motives and ongoing risk (Fauman and Fauman, 1981). Possible motivations include manipulation, revenge, a desire to join a dead relative, or response to a command hallucination. Because patients who have attempted suicide are likely to try again, ascertain whether the patient has had previous suicidal thoughts and the duration of these thoughts. The patient's attitude toward surviving the attempt is also important. The patient may be relieved or angry, fearful of retaliation by parents or relatives, or frightened or complacent about the attempt.

Also explore factors in the patient's life that may have led to the suicide attempt. Common stressors associated with self-destructive behavior include relationships, especially with parents or caregivers; changes within the family; illness; school problems; peer pressure; trouble with the law; trauma, such as incest, rape, or physical abuse; and substance abuse.

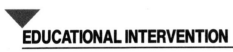

PHARMACOLOGIC INTERVENTION

Unless the patient is acutely psychotic or agitated, pharmacologic intervention is not needed. However, if the patient suffers from an acute organic psychosis (such as toxic, metabolic, or infectious encephalopathy), the clinician must take specific measures to treat the underlying medical illness. A psychotic patient may require haloperidol (Haldol) 0.05 to 0.15 mg/kg/day in two or three divided doses or chlorpromazine (Thorazine) 0.1 mg/kg every 4 to 6 hours. A nonpsychotic but agitated patient can be given hydroxyzine (Vistaril) 0.2 mg/kg or diphenhydramine (Benadryl) 5 mg/kg/day in four divided doses. Benzodiazepines should not be given because of the possible adverse effect of these drugs on attention deficit disorder and because of the potential for addiction. Some evidence indicates that lorazepam (Ativan) is safe to use in children and adolescents. Lorazepam may be appropriate for managing nonpsychotic agitation even when antihistamines are contraindicated because of their anticholinergic properties.

EDUCATIONAL INTERVENTION

Never blame family members for the patient's self-destructive behavior. Instead, support their attempts to cope with and listen to the child. Share with them any information obtained from the patient, including possible reasons for his behavior, so that a dialogue can develop between the child and the parents. Additionally, work closely with the parents to suggest ways of ensuring the child's safety at home, such as removing drugs and weapons from easily accessible locations, providing more supervision, and devoting more uninterrupted time to the child.

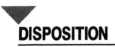

DISPOSITION

The disposition varies, depending on the parents' responsiveness to your requests. If the parents appear genuinely willing to comply, you can discharge the patient to their care, although you should ensure that the patient continues to receive help by giving the parents phone numbers to call in case of an emergency and by arranging a follow-up appointment with an outpatient therapist for the next day.

If the parents have difficulty responding to the instructions or if the safety of the patient is in doubt, consider hospitalizing the patient, finding another family member with whom the patient can temporarily reside, or, in extreme cases, placing the patient in emergency foster care.

Safety is the overriding consideration in the disposition of the suicidal child or adolescent. Hospitalize a patient with a psychosis, drug or alcohol addiction, organic mental syndrome, or any serious condition resulting in depression. Those who have no will to live or who refuse to accept or comply with an outpatient appointment should also be hospitalized. In addition, whenever the patient demonstrates suicidal intent, either hospitalize the patient or refer him to a residential crisis intervention center.

▼ MEDICOLEGAL CONSIDERATIONS

In many states, the standard for civil commitment is whether the minor is "in need of psychiatric care that cannot be provided in a less restrictive setting," which is less stringent than the adult standard of "dangerousness."

Children younger than the age of consent can be signed into a hospital without the need for commitment procedures. However, parents or guardians may want the child released against medical advice. In such cases, determine if state laws permit the detention of the patient via commitment. If the patient was injured "accidentally" (for instance, by ingesting drugs or alcohol or by using a firearm), the parents may be liable for child neglect. Keep in mind that a clinician has a duty to report instances of neglect to the state child protective agency and to take necessary precautions to ensure the child's safety.

IDENTIFYING THE PROBLEM: VIOLENT BEHAVIOR

Juvenile violence is increasing at nearly twice the rate of adult violence. Suicide and homicide account for the greatest number of deaths in adolescents and for the greatest number of emergency psychiatric visits in this population (Rosenn, 1984). Violent behavior in children and adolescents ranges from behavioral dyscontrol to premeditated homicide. In some cases, violent youth have little if any psychopathology; in other cases, they may be profoundly mentally disturbed. Violence in young persons, except in self-defense, should be considered pathological until proven otherwise. Very young children may be unaware of the seriousness of their attack on another person. Yet all homicidal behavior signifies a breakdown in communication and the containment of thoughts and feelings. The younger the child, the more likely that he has a serious personality disorder or is the victim of parental abuse or neglect.

Thoroughly examine any child or adolescent who has an immediate history of harming or threatening to harm someone or destroy property. The evaluation may be complicated by the need to control the patient while establishing sufficient trust to enable the patient to reveal the details of the event and his attendant feelings and thoughts. Because the patient may not be fully aware of the events that just occurred or may deliberately withhold or distort information, interview those who accompanied the patient to the ED to obtain a complete picture of the episode. Depending on the perceived seriousness and awareness of the act, the patient's emotions can be intense. An increasingly frequent contributing factor in youthful violence is drug and alcohol intoxication or withdrawal.

Mental status findings

Examine the patient to assess his recall of and emotional reaction to the event, use of drugs or alcohol, level of intellectual functioning, possible stressors (such as loss of a significant relationship), history of psychiatric illness or psychosis, and history of child abuse. Furthermore, you must ascertain the parents' reaction to the violent behavior. Although violence in children usually represents a communication failure among family members, a newly violent child or adolescent requires careful screening for medical and acute psychiatric causes. Aggressively homicidal youth may insist that the act was an accident or done in self-defense.

Physical findings
Conduct a physical examination to rule out underlying medical problems that result in violent behavior. In particular, be alert for impaired consciousness, orientation, and intellectual functioning; physical handicaps; signs of physical or sexual abuse; specific neurologic impairment; symptoms of intoxication or withdrawal; and any other signs of acute medical illness, such as infection.

Differential diagnosis
You must rule out depression and look for signs of physical or sexual abuse (see *Signs of physical and sexual abuse*). Violent behavior may also be associated with alcohol or drug intoxication or withdrawal and organic mental states, which can impair reality testing, impulse control, and judgment.

SIGNS OF PHYSICAL AND SEXUAL ABUSE

Physical abuse
- Multiple injuries at various stages of healing
- Bruises in the pattern of finger marks or strap marks
- Burns from cigarettes
- Scalding injuries
- Bite marks
- Bald spots (from hair pulling)
- Injuries of the long bones, especially dislocated metaphyses or epiphyses, spiral fractures, or subperiosteal thickening
- Rupture of viscera

Sexual abuse
- Genital or anal tears, bruises or irritations, discharge, and sexually transmitted disease
- Encopresis (associated with anal rape)
- Enuresis (from regression, overexcitation, or fears related to sexual abuse)
- Psychosomatic symptoms, such as headaches or stomachaches

Source: Robinson, 1986. Adapted with permission of the publisher.

INTERPERSONAL INTERVENTION

An acutely agitated, angry, and violent patient must be prevented from harming himself or others. Although the patient may be out of control and frightened, the clinician must maintain a nonjudgmental, calm, and firm attitude and treat the patient with respect. Sometimes patients can be controlled by removing them from the family, placing them in a quiet room, attending to their basic needs, or providing food and support. In other cases, mild physical or four-point restraint (restraining the arms and legs with padded leather straps) or the presence of many staff members may be needed to convince the patient that he is in a protected setting. Until a diagnosis is established, physically restraining a violent youth is safer than using sedation; drugs may contribute to an inaccurate diagnosis or worsen an underlying organic condition.

PHARMACOLOGIC INTERVENTION

When physical restraint fails to calm an agitated patient and medical causes of the anxiety are ruled out, the clinician can quiet the patient by administering hydroxyzine 0.2 mg/kg I.M. or orally or diphenhydramine 5 mg/kg for 24 hours in four divided doses. For a more acutely agitated patient in whom no medical causes can be found, the physician can safely use either chlorpromazine 0.1 mg/kg every 4 to 6 hours or haloperidol 0.05 to 0.15 mg/kg/day in two or three divided doses.

In almost no case should the clinician use benzodiazepines or other secondary and tertiary anti-aggressive drugs, such as lithium (Eskalith), carbamazepine (Tegretol), or propranolol (Inderal), during emergency management of violent behavior. Benzodiazepines carry the risk of further disinhibiting aggressive behavior, especially when the patient has a coexistent attention deficit disorder, such as hyperactivity (although benzodiazepines may be indicated for alcohol or sedative withdrawal syndromes). The other drugs have a long onset of action, and they could not be administered safely without further baseline medical studies and a more precise diagnosis.

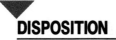

DISPOSITION

After assessing the seriousness of the violence, arriving at a diagnosis, and judging the appropriateness and potential success of the parental response, evaluate the risk of continued violent behavior. Potentially homicidal children and adolescents considered at high risk for violence share one or more of the following characteristics: neurologic impairment, schizophrenia, underlying psychiatric illness, limited intellectual functioning, school failure, poor family situation, personal experience with brutality, history of fire setting or cruelty to animals, conduct-disordered behavior at an early age, labile and highly anxious or angry affect, and action-oriented personality. They may also believe that killing is an acceptable way to express anger, have access to a weapon, or have a homicidal plan (Rosenn, 1984).

If a primary medical or psychiatric condition is causing the violent behavior, initiate treatment, which probably entails hospitalizing the patient. When multiple causes are involved, intervene with a combination of medical treatment, psychological support, containment of dangerous behavior, and immediate crisis intervention. If protective pharmacologic or physical restraint is needed to ensure that no harm comes to the patient or staff, a short-term inpatient evaluation is probably necessary.

If the patient is discharged in parental custody, the clinician should provide emergency phone numbers and schedule an outpatient appointment for the following day. Because a homicidal child can quickly become a suicidal one, parents should be familiar with the signs of depression and remorse, which may indicate a possible suicide attempt.

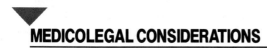

MEDICOLEGAL CONSIDERATIONS

The clinician can legally commit a minor patient who is mentally disturbed or dangerous to persons or property. However, voluntary hospitalization or parental consent can often be obtained instead.

IDENTIFYING THE PROBLEM: RUNAWAY BEHAVIOR

Most youths run away to escape a destructive home life. They do not run away simply to join another person or family or to have a different life-style. Before puberty, boys run away twice as often as girls, but after puberty, girls leave home two to three times more frequently than boys (Rosenn, 1984). Most adolescents who run away are never seen for psychiatric evaluation. Yet running away is not necessarily evidence of psychopathology; the child may be reacting to a pathological family situation (Stierlin and Ravenscroft, 1972; Stierlin, 1973).

Some runaway children or adolescents come to the ED alone; others are brought by their parents after they have returned home or are suspected of planning to leave home. Sometimes parents come alone to the emergency service for help a day or several days after the child has left. The parents may be angry, guilty, grief stricken, or fearful and may need advice on coping with the event.

Abortive runaways (those who have unsuccessfully escaped from home) usually return through their own efforts. For example, they may feign an illness that results in an ED visit or may turn themselves into the police. *Schizoidal runaways* are the most psychiatrically disturbed and usually break down away from home. Their psychotic symptoms or depression may bring them to the ED in a crisis. *Casual runaways* separate easily from the home and rarely come to the ED unless they want to manipulate their parents or guardians. Because they are socially and sexually precocious, casual runaways survive the runaway culture well. In contrast, *crisis runaways* remain preoccupied with the family even after being away for days or weeks. These runaways may come to the ED as a result of aggressive, sexual, or antisocial behavior they have displayed to carry out some unconscious "mission" of the parents (such as fighting with someone whom the parents intensely dislike).

Mental status findings

When conducting the mental status examination, look for signs of psychosis or idiosyncratic and bizarre thinking, panic, depression or suicidal ideas, remorse, guilt, ambivalence about returning home, and fear of reprisal. In taking the patient's history, note whether the patient exhibits endangering behavior, which increases the likelihood of exploitation by others, and assess his use of alcohol or drugs, promiscuity, or antisocial activity. In addition, gather details about the runaway event itself: the patient's motivation for leaving; contact with parents while away; living arrangements and survival tactics; length of time away; reason for coming to the ED; whether the runaway was planned or impulsive; whether the patient remained alone or with a group; and whether this event was an isolated incident or part of a chronic problem.

Physical findings

The physical examination supports or refutes data from the patient's history. Look for injuries (bruises, lacerations, welts, scratches), malnutrition, signs of assault (both physical and sexual), and alcohol or drug abuse.

Laboratory studies

Findings may warrant a chest X-ray, complete blood count and differential, urine drug screen, and a hepatic and renal profile, including electrolytes, glucose, and blood urea nitrogen.

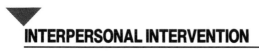

INTERPERSONAL INTERVENTION

Begin to establish a rapport with the patient while assessing his physical health. A nonjudgmental and concerned approach facilitates the development of a relationship. Rapport is essential for gaining the youth's trust in order to learn more about the family problems that caused the runaway behavior.

The primary goal is to determine whether to send the patient home immediately. If the patient is psychotic, suicidal, medically ill, or physically or sexually abused, hospitalization is necessary. If the patient is ambivalent about returning home and has no indications for hospitalization, the clinician becomes the key to reuniting the parents and child. To prevent the patient from leaving the emergency setting, carefully assess the patient's fears, ambivalence, and possible negative consequences of returning home before contacting the parents.

▼
DISPOSITION

Before discharging the patient, arrange a meeting between the parents and the youth in the ED. If the patient's health or safety is at stake, hospitalize the patient and then notify the parents.

▼
MEDICOLEGAL CONSIDERATIONS

Never discharge a minor without informing the parents of the youth's whereabouts and condition and without obtaining their consent. If you determine that the patient should be placed outside the home, the parents must be involved in this decision, even if only temporary placement is necessary. States laws delineate *in loco parentis* responsibilities for caregivers of youths under age 18.

The term *emancipated minor* describes an adolescent who has obtained the legal right to live independently from parents or guardians. Emancipated minors do not usually have other adult rights and responsibilities. Be alert for adolescents who declare themselves emancipated out of desire rather than because of legal status. An adolescent who lives alone or has a child is more likely to be legally emancipated. If you cannot determine the patient's status, you must notify the parents or other concerned relatives of the disposition plans.

▼
IDENTIFYING THE PROBLEM: CHILD ABUSE

Child abuse comprises all forms of adult behavior that are physically or psychologically destructive to a child's well-being and normal growth and development. Up to 4 million cases of child abuse occur in the United States every year, and as many as 2,000 children die each year as a result of abuse (Ludwig, 1983). Abuse may recur within families and is seen in all socioeconomic and ethnic groups. (See *Risk factors for child abuse,* page 208.) Because child abuse is always a family crisis, any childhood emergency should arouse the examiner's suspicion. Become familiar with child abuse laws and reporting practices and with hospital and community resources.

RISK FACTORS FOR CHILD ABUSE

The child
- Infants and preschoolers
- Medical problems
- Mental retardation
- Physical handicap
- Neurological impairment
- Hyperactivity
- Prolonged hospitalization during infancy

The families
- Lack of preparation for parenting
- Poor role models
- Use of corporal punishment
- Unrealistic expectations for the child
- Severe social isolation
- Critical extended family
- Severe parental conflict

Parent-child interaction
- Economic problems
- Unemployment
- Crowding and poor housing
- Parental illness

The parents
- Impulse disorders
- Drug or alcohol abuse
- Psychiatric illness
- Abused as a child

Source: Sargent et al., 1984. Robinson, 1986.

The clinician must intervene in a sensitive and professional manner in this highly complex and intense family emergency.

Types of child abuse

The clinician should be familiar with the four types of child abuse (Sargent et al., 1984):

Physical abuse. Abuse that results in physical injury, including fractures, burns, bruises, or internal damage. Physical abuse may be disguised as discipline or punishment and accounts for about 65% of reported child abuse cases.

Sexual abuse. Any contact or interaction between a child and an adult when the child is used for the sexual stimulation of the abuser. Sexual abuse may also be committed by a minor who is older than or in a position of power over the child. This type of abuse accounts for about 20% of all reported cases.

Child neglect. Acts of omission, such as the failure of a parent to provide for a child's welfare, basic needs, and proper level of care with respect to food, clothing, shelter, hygiene, medical attention, or supervision. Child neglect is seen in about 10% of all reported cases.

Emotional abuse. Abuse that results in impaired psychological growth and development of the child. Verbal abuse and excessive demands on a child's performance are forms of emotional persecution that can result in a negative self-image and disturbed behavior. Emotional abuse accounts for about 5% of all reported cases, although it almost always accompanies other forms of abuse.

Because child abuse is rarely the chief complaint, be alert to evidence of abuse when examining the child. For example, physical abuse is likely if the injured child was not brought to the ED promptly or if the history is inconsistent; includes repeated injury or hospitalization, family stress, or preexisting illness in the child; or does not adequately explain the circumstances of the injury.

Sexual abuse is a possibility when a prepubertal girl has gynecological symptoms or when the patient is sexually preoccupied, reveals stories with a sexual content, or has a history of abrupt changes in behavior or school performance. The patient may reveal incidents of sexual abuse purposely or accidentally. Disclosure always precipitates a crisis for the family.

Child neglect becomes apparent when examining the child for other problems. Parents who neglect their children may underestimate or overestimate their child's physical and emotional needs. Children with "failure to thrive" or developmental delay, if nonorganically based, are products of neglect. The feeding, growth, and developmental history provide clues to neglect.

Mental status findings

A younger child may be fearful, have unreasonable expectations (such as a reunion with a perfect family or an undoing of the abuse), be overly responsible, have a difficult temperament with impulsivity and mood swings, or be shy and withdrawn. The younger patient may have nightmares or night terrors, cling and whine, and refuse to stay with a particular person. An older child may be hypersexual and promiscuous, exhibit deviant sexual behavior, run away, abuse alcohol or drugs, or attempt suicide.

Physical findings

Signs of abuse can be seen in the skin, hair, eyes, ears, bones, central nervous system, gastrointestinal system, and genitourinary system.

Laboratory studies

Laboratory studies to evaluate abuse include a bone survey; urethral, vaginal, oral, and anal cultures and wet mounts; pregnancy test; clotting factors; computed tomography scan or magnetic resonance imaging; abdominal flatplate X-ray; and urinalysis.

▼
INTERPERSONAL INTERVENTION

Intervention begins during the first contact with the child and family. The clinician must be thoughtful, sensitive, goal-directed, and action-oriented. The clinician's objective is to protect the health and well-being of the child and to provide as much consistency in the child's life as possible.

A clinician who suspects child abuse may have strong feelings of anger for the abuser and sympathy for the victim. Even so, the clinician must attempt to form a satisfactory relationship with the child and parents. A confrontational and accusatory approach is inappropriate and will frighten both the patient and family members. The child's fear and concerns for his parents should be respected. The clinician should convey to the parents an understanding of their emotional state and reaction to their child without condoning or sanctioning the abusive behavior. Management of child abuse should include a consultation with other members of the psychosocial team to validate suspicions and determine the disposition.

PHARMACOLOGIC INTERVENTION

The use of medication for a victim of child abuse should be avoided unless absolutely necessary. Pharmacologic intervention further confirms the child's fear that he is sick, bad, or out of control and can increase the child's sense of victimization.

EDUCATIONAL INTERVENTION

Once a diagnosis of abuse is made, the clinician must inform the parents and, without equivocation, describe the follow-up plans. Their response to this information may supply additional corroborating or refuting data. Families who cooperate early in the evaluation are more easily helped.

DISPOSITION

The disposition should be guided by a concern for the child's safety and by legal constraints (see "Medicolegal considerations" below). Hospitalization is necessary when the child's physical or mental status warrants it or when the clinician is concerned about the child's safety at home.

MEDICOLEGAL CONSIDERATIONS

The clinician must file two child abuse reports—by telephone to the child abuse hotline and on a legal form documenting the detailed findings of the examination. The child abuse agency should be contacted immediately to provide further assistance in implementing a treatment plan for the child and family. Ultimate disposition of the child outside the hospital is the legal domain of the child abuse agency.

In most cases, if the child remains at risk, the agency must complete a full evaluation of the situation within 24 hours. Sometimes the examining physician must provide courtroom testimony. In other cases, the clinician may need to involve the hospital administration or legal authorities to protect the child, hospitalize the child, or remove threatening and violent family members.

In all cases, family members should be informed of their rights and responsibilities, which include a full court hearing with legal representation and a continued duty to protect the child's well-being. The clinician should explain that, if the parents cooperate with medical, legal, and psychiatric authorities, the child can be returned to their custody.

IDENTIFYING THE PROBLEM: ALCOHOL AND DRUG ABUSE

Alcohol and drug abuse are prevalent among younger persons and increasingly part of all adolescent emergencies. The clinician should suspect drug intoxication or withdrawal in all cases of acute changes in the patient's mental state. Substance abuse should be part of the differential diagnosis in every emergency evaluation of children and adolescents.

Drugs and alcohol alter perceptions; alter the speed, content, and coherence of thought; diminish insight; and impair judgment. Indeed, these substances can have a substantial impact on youthful behavior and can cause psychiatric emergencies that might not otherwise occur. In assessing an adolescent, the clinician must obtain a detailed drug history, including the duration of drug abuse, the type and quantity of drugs used, and the perceived effects on the patient.

The clinician should not be misled by a history of substance abuse into erroneously assuming that alcohol or drug abuse is the predominant problem. Many adolescents with major psychiatric disorders, such as schizophrenia, mania, or depression, self-medicate with drugs and alcohol. Consequently, the clinician must conduct a comprehensive medical, neurologic, and psychiatric evaluation before making a final diagnosis and treatment decision.

See Chapter 4, Alcohol Emergencies, and Chapter 5, Drug Abuse Emergencies, for more detailed information on relevant interventions, dispositions, and medicolegal considerations.

REFERENCES

Fauman, B., and Fauman, M. *Emergency Psychiatry for the House Officer.* Baltimore: Williams and Wilkins, 1981.

Khan, A.V. *Psychiatric Emergencies on Pediatrics.* Chicago: Yearbook Medical Publications, 1979.

Ludwig, S. "Child Abuse," in *Textbook of Pediatric Emergency Medicine.* Edited by Fleichen, G., et al. Baltimore: Williams and Wilkins, 1983.

Pfeffer, C.R. "Suicidal Behavior of Children: A Review with Implications for Research and Practice," *American Journal of Psychiatry* 138(2):154-159, February 1981.

Robinson, J. "Emergencies I," in *Manual of Clinical Child Psychiatry.* Edited by Robson, K. Washington, D.C.: APA Press, Inc., 1986.

Rosenn, D.W. "Psychiatric Emergencies in Children and Adolescents," in *Emergency Psychiatry: Concepts, Methods, and Practices.* Edited by Bassuk, E.L., and Birk, A.W. New York: Plenum Press, 1984.

Sargent, J., et al. "Crisis Intervention in Children and Adolescents," in *Psychiatric Emergencies.* Edited by Dubin, W., et al. New York: Churchill Livingstone, 1984.

Stierlin, H. "A Family Perspective on Adolescent Runaways," *Archives of General Psychiatry* 29:56-62, 1973.

Stierlin, H., and Ravenscroft, K. "Varieties of Adolescent 'Separation Conflicts.'" *British Journal of Medical Psychology* 45(4):299-313, December 1972.

14

GERIATRIC EMERGENCIES

Psychiatric emergencies involving elderly persons can occur in a crisis center, emergency department (ED), medical-surgical unit, nursing home, or private residence. Because psychiatric disorders are prevalent in older persons (Jenike, 1985; Minden, 1984; Walker and Covington, 1984), the clinician should be familiar with the typical signs of mental disturbance in this population. This chapter focuses on psychiatric disorders that can appear differently in elderly persons than in younger persons and on disorders unique to geriatric patients.

IDENTIFYING THE PROBLEM: DEMENTIA

Dementia is a general term for the chronic organic mental disorder that causes loss of intellectual and other higher brain functions. Nearly 40% of those with dementia have treatable or reversible forms (Thompson, 1987). Unfortunately, the term is frequently misused as a synonym for Alzheimer's disease, which can lead to pessimism and passivity among clinicians.

Since dementia itself is not a crisis, the clinician's role is to identify the undiagnosed demented patient, treat presenting problems (such as delirium or psychosis), initiate physical examinations and laboratory studies, and counsel the patient's family.

The patient with dementia is usually brought to the emergency setting by a relative or caregiver. Typical chief complaints include confusion, disorientation, or wandering; inappropriate social behavior; anxiety or depression; delusions (for example, that others are stealing from the patient); or verbal or physical aggression.

Mental status findings

As described in the *DSM-III-R* (1987), major findings in dementia are impaired memory, abstract thinking, and judgment and disruption of higher cortical function. Although both short- and long-term memory are affected, short-term memory loss usually occurs first. A patient with an impaired short-term memory is unable to learn new information, such as recalling three objects after five minutes. Long-term memory deficits are characterized by a loss of recall for past events, such as birthplace, occupation, and well-known dates. Mild memory loss is part of normal aging and not considered dementia.

Patients who are unable to find similarities between words or concepts have impaired abstract thinking. They may also have difficulty in defining previously known words. Impaired judgment is apparent when the patient is unable to make reasonable plans for interpersonal, family, financial, or occupational issues. An impairment in social judgment can lead to inappropriate or disinhibited behavior, such as disrobing in public. Disruption of higher cortical function manifests as aphasia (impairment in receptive or expressive language), apraxia (impairment in purposive motor acts), agnosia (failure to recognize objects, body parts, or persons), or constructional problems (such as an inability to copy a figure on paper).

In conducting the mental status examination, the clinician should use a structured rating instrument (see Appendix C: Folstein Mini-Mental State Examination).

Physical findings

Although no specific guidelines exist for the physical examination of a patient with dementia, conduct a thorough physical and neurologic evaluation to rule out the diverse causes of the disorder.

Laboratory studies

The laboratory evaluation of patients with dementia is extensive: a complete blood count (CBC), electrolyte and glucose levels, hepatic and renal profiles, urinalysis, thyroid profile, syphilis screen, urinary corticosteroids, erythrocyte sedimentation rate, lupus profile, human immunodeficiency virus antibody titer, chest X-ray, and electrocardiogram (ECG). Also order neurologic studies, such as a computed tomography (CT) scan or magnetic resonance imaging, lumbar puncture, and electroencephalogram. Some of these studies can be initiated in the emergency setting while arrangements for hospitalization or other care are made.

Differential diagnosis

The differential diagnosis of dementia is lengthy and cannot be completed in the ED. However, since many causes of dementia are treatable (see *Treatable causes of dementia*), the clinician should focus on ruling out life-threatening causes, such as tumor, infection, and hematoma.

Dementia, a chronic and stable condition that is not accompanied by clouded consciousness, must be differentiated from delirium, an acute illness that causes altered consciousness.

Major depression can resemble dementia. Complaints of impaired memory, thinking, and concentration and an overall decrease in function are consistent with depression-induced dementia, or pseudodementia (Wells, 1979). Unlike a typical dementia, such as Alzheimer's disease, depression-induced dementia has a rapid onset and commonly occurs in patients with histories of depression or bipolar disorder. The pseudodemented patient is more likely than the organically demented patient to complain of memory loss and is also more likely to answer "I don't know" to questions. A timely diagnosis of depression can avert a misdiagnosis of irreversible dementia in an otherwise treatable patient.

INTERPERSONAL INTERVENTION

Place a patient with dementia in a quiet, well-lighted room, supervised by family or staff members to prevent wandering or accidental injury. Explain the treatment plan to the patient, and avoid

TREATABLE CAUSES OF DEMENTIA

Cardiac disease
(arrhythmias, congestive heart failure, myocardial infarction)

Pulmonary disease
(chronic obstructive pulmonary disease, pulmonary emboli)

Hepatic disease
(cirrhosis, hepatitis, Wilson's disease)

Renal disease
(urinary tract infection that worsens mild nephritis, dehydration)

Vascular disease
(subdural hematoma, cerebrovascular accident)

Infection

Endocrine disease
(hypothyroidism, Cushing's syndrome, Addison's disease, diabetes, hypoglycemia)

Electrolyte imbalance
(hyponatremia, hypernatremia, hypercalcemia)

Vitamin deficiencies
(thiamine, niacin, riboflavin, folate, ascorbic acid, vitamin A, vitamin B_{12})

Drugs
(alcohol, tranquilizers, over-the-counter drugs, prescription medications)

Exogenous toxins
(carbon monoxide, bromide, mercury, lead)

Tumors

Normal pressure hydrocephalus

Depression

subjecting him to multiple interviews. Demented patients need re-assurance from a supportive clinician.

PHARMACOLOGIC INTERVENTION

Demented patients may be agitated or psychotic. Such patients can be treated with small doses of a neuroleptic agent, such as haloperidol (Haldol) 1 to 2 mg or thiothixene (Navane) 2 to 5 mg orally or I.M. Medications with strong anticholinergic side effects should not be prescribed because they can induce delirium. The clinician should also avoid benzodiazepines, which may cause excessive sedation or exacerbate confusion.

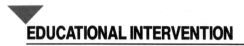

EDUCATIONAL INTERVENTION

Education is an unrealistic goal for a demented patient in the emergency setting. Family members, however, are an integral part of subsequent care and should receive information on the patient's condition. Unless the cause of the dementia has been previously established, do not assume that the patient has Alzheimer's disease. Explain to the family that Alzheimer's disease is diagnosed by eliminating other dementias, and help them understand that their continued help is essential.

If a treatable cause of dementia is found, reassure the family that the patient does not have Alzheimer's disease. If the dementia is caused by poor self-care (such as malnutrition), the family must make appropriate arrangements for the patient's care.

The diagnosis of an irreversible dementia, such as Alzheimer's disease, is devastating for the patient's family, who will need support and guidance. Discuss such issues as power of attorney and nursing home placement. In addition, refer the relatives to a support group for spouses and family members of Alzheimer's disease victims. Families should know that the patient's angry outbursts, uncharacteristic profanity, and forgetfulness are not willful but part of the progressing disease.

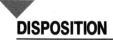

DISPOSITION

Given the serious prognosis of dementia, most patients should be hospitalized for a thorough evaluation. Based on the patient's condition and the family's cooperation, anticipate the posthospital disposition by determining whether the family members are willing to continue to keep the patient in their home. Relatives may take a patient to the ED because they are "burnt out" and can no longer care for the patient. In such cases, suggest that the patient live with another relative or in a nursing facility.

▼
MEDICOLEGAL CONSIDERATIONS

Patients with grossly impaired judgment and diminished intellect may be clinically incompetent. Such patients are unable to participate in medical, legal, or financial decisions. In assessing the competence of the demented patient, ask several questions:

• Is the patient oriented to time, place, person, and circumstances?
• Does the patient acknowledge a problem?
• Is the patient willing to be treated?
• If the patient refuses treatment, does he understand the consequences?

A disoriented person is unlikely to be competent. Yet refusing treatment does not indicate that the patient is incompetent and must be weighed against other mental status features. Clinicians can legally provide emergency treatment for clinically incompetent patients. However, the clinician should obtain consent from family members or a legal guardian as soon as the crisis is over.

▼
IDENTIFYING THE PROBLEM: DELIRIUM

Delirium in geriatric patients is an acute organic mental disorder with potentially serious consequences. Rapid recognition and reversal of the condition are critical. The essential feature of delirium is a sudden change in behavior. In interpreting the patient's history (which is always obtained from a relative or friend), the clinician must be aware that delirium may be more subtle in an elderly person than in a younger adult. Elderly patients commonly have a "quiet" delirium, which manifests as a loss of interest and concentration but actually represents a change in consciousness. Clues to a diagnosis of delirium are rapid deterioration in behavior or orientation, preexisting dementia, recent infection or head injury, recent change in medication, and new neurologic signs.

Dementia and delirium can coexist; delirium may develop in demented patients as a result of an infection or drug side effect.

The clinician should focus on changes in the patient's daily routine, environment, and medical and drug status that occurred about the same time as the change in behavior.

Use of over-the-counter (OTC) drugs or alcohol is also associated with delirium. Many older patients do not perceive OTC preparations as drugs. When questioning the patient, be sure to ask, "Do you buy any medicines off the shelf in the drugstore for sleep, colds, arthritis, or other problems?" Similarly, the elderly patient may not believe that drinking can be harmful or may deny drinking. Many elderly persons sip sherry, wine, or cordials daily, which can lead to alcohol withdrawal if they are hospitalized for a medical-surgical problem. Encourage family members to report the elderly patient's use of alcohol and prescription or OTC drugs. If possible, they should bring in all the patient's medications for evaluation.

An elderly patient who takes one or more drugs with anticholinergic (atropine-like) properties is susceptible to central anticholinergic syndrome. Signs and symptoms of this delirious state include dry skin and mucosae, blurred vision, constipation, urine retention, tachycardia, dilated and unreactive pupils, and flushed facies. In severe cases, the patient may have seizures, hyperreflexia, fever, slurred speech, and ataxia. Commonly used medications with anticholinergic effects include hypnotics, such as scopolamine (Transderm-V); eye drops, such as atropine (Atroposol), scopolamine (Buscospan), and cyclopentolate (Cyclogyl); antihistamines, such as diphenhydramine (Benadryl), hydroxyzine (Atarax), chlorpheniramine (Chlor-Trimeton), and promethazine (Pentazine); antiparkinsonian agents, such as benztropine (Cogentin) and trihexyphenidyl (Trihexane); tricyclic antidepressants, such as amitriptyline (Elavil), nortriptyline (Aventyl), imipramine (Tofranil), and doxepin (Sinequan); and neuroleptic agents, such as chlorpromazine (Thorazine), thioridazine (Mellaril), and mesoridazine (Serentil).

Mental status findings
Typical mental status findings in a delirious elderly patient include disorientation, disturbed sleep-wake cycle, clouding of consciousness, visual hallucinations, illusions, delusions, fluctuating symptoms, agitation, and impaired attention, concentration, and memory.

Physical findings

Although delirium does not cause any specific physical symptoms, relevant findings include scalp lacerations or contusions, signs of hypoxemia ("dusty" skin color or blue nailbeds), fever, increased heart rate (greater than 100 beats/minute), and increased respiratory rate (greater than 30 breaths/minute).

The emergence of new neurologic signs – tremors, paralyses, asymmetrical or abnormal reflexes, ocular signs, or aphasia – should immediately trigger a consultation with a neurologist and appropriate diagnostic tests, especially a CT scan. (See Chapter 3, Delirium, for additional physical findings and their interpretation.)

Laboratory studies

The minimum standard laboratory evaluation of the delirious elderly patient includes blood glucose, electrolyte, and blood urea nitrogen levels; CBC and differential; serum levels of all drugs; ECG; urinalysis; chest X-ray; and arterial blood gas analysis. If these tests are negative, order a lumbar puncture and CT scan.

Differential diagnosis

Because delirium can coexist with dementia, be especially alert for changes in the patient's mental status. When evaluating the patient for the first time, rely on family members to supply the mental status history. A sudden deterioration in mental status should not immediately be ascribed to dementia alone; do not overlook readily reversible causes of delirium, such as urinary tract infection.

▼ INTERPERSONAL INTERVENTION

The primary intervention is assuring the delirious elderly patient that the condition will pass. The clinician should also conduct frequent orientation and reality checks and involve the patient's family members (familiar faces can help orient the patient). If the patient is combative or agitated, physical restraint (such as a Posey vest) may be needed to prevent self-harm or harm to others. Restraints may also be necessary to ensure that the patient does not disconnect intravenous lines or other equipment.

▼
PHARMACOLOGIC INTERVENTION

While investigating the cause of the delirium, the clinician may need to administer psychotropic medication to treat the patient's behavioral symptoms. The clinician must avoid further compromising the patient's brain function, which can occur, for example, when chlorpromazine is given to a patient with anticholinergic delirium. Any psychotropic drugs given to delirious patients should be short-acting and relatively free of anticholinergic side effects. Benzodiazepines should not be prescribed for elderly patients with impaired consciousness; these drugs further impair cortical function. To calm a highly agitated patient, the clinician can administer a 1-mg dose of haloperidol I.M. Other high-potency neuroleptic agents can also be used, including fluphenazine (Prolixin) 1 mg, trifluoperazine (Stelazine) 2 mg, and thiothixene 2 mg. These doses can be repeated every 2 hours. Although any psychotropic drug can depress brain function, neuroleptic agents can also cause extrapyramidal symptoms. Other pharmacologic interventions are based solely on the diagnosis (for example, to correct an electrolyte or acid-base imbalance).

Delirium caused by anticholinergic drugs is a medical emergency. Treat patients who have anticholinergic delirium with physostigmine (Antilirium) 1 to 2 mg I.V. (slow push) or I.M. (Dubin et al., 1986). Since physostigmine's duration of action is 2 hours, the dose can be repeated at 2-hour intervals, or more frequently if needed. Overly aggressive treatment can precipitate a cholinergic crisis, which can be reversed with atropine 0.5 mg for each 1 mg of physostigmine (Hall et al., 1981). Additional complications of physostigmine treatment are vomiting, hypotension, and seizures.

▼
EDUCATIONAL INTERVENTION

The patient's family or caregiver may benefit from advice about the prevention of drug-induced delirium. Tell them to inform the primary care physician about the patient's use of OTC medications and to monitor the drugs he takes. Advise them to encourage the elderly person to avoid alcohol, and teach them the early signs of mental status changes.

▼
DISPOSITION

Most delirious elderly patients should be hospitalized for further treatment and evaluation. However, a patient with a transitory, drug-induced delirium can be discharged to the care of family or friends if they schedule a follow-up appointment with the primary care physician. Make reasonable efforts to return the patient to his former environment (Minden, 1984).

▼
MEDICOLEGAL CONSIDERATIONS

Most delirious patients are legally incompetent. However, before initiating treatment or ordering restraints, try to obtain consent from a family member. If such consent cannot be obtained, a second clinical opinion (documented in the medical record) and notification of relatives will suffice.

▼
IDENTIFYING THE PROBLEM: ADJUSTMENT DISORDERS

Adjustment disorders, usually characterized by anxiety and depression, can have an organic, psychodynamic, or psychosocial cause (Goodstein, 1985). To avoid deterioration of the elderly patient who has acute problems in living, institute rapid and appropriate intervention. Some elderly patients have anxiety or depressive symptoms. Others have an increase in bodily complaints, disturbed sleep, problems in concentration and thinking clearly, and forgetfulness or difficulty recalling words.

The key concepts in assessing adjustment disorders in geriatric persons are *loss* and *change.* Losses can be physical (diminished vision), personal (death of spouse), occupational or financial (retirement), or symbolic (loss of youth). Changes can also precipitate emotional difficulties, especially a change in residence. A move to a nursing home can be traumatic even for a well-adjusted older person.

Preexisting dementia, such as Alzheimer's disease, exacerbates the adjustment disorder, yet transitory disorders are treatable. A patient should not be disregarded because of a preexisting dementia nor should all emotional symptoms be attributed to "senility" (Goodstein, 1985).

Mental status findings

In addition to the usual clinical signs of anxiety and depression, elderly patients (especially those with mild cognitive impairment) may respond to loss or change with apathy, irritability, bodily complaints (pain, disability, constipation), faulty memory, inattention, hopelessness, and paranoia. Also, look for signs of suicidal thoughts or self-destructive behavior. Elderly persons who have physical disabilities or who live alone are at particularly high risk for suicide (Goodstein, 1985; Minden, 1984). Warning signs of suicidal intent include apathy, hopelessness, poor self-care, noncompliance with essential medications, and decreased social contacts.

Physical findings

Adjustment disorder symptoms are commonly related to deterioration of the patient's physical condition. Therefore, check the patient's vision, hearing, dentition, joint mobility, bladder and bowel function, and (in men) sexual potency. The presence of infections or a change in nervous system response must also be determined.

Laboratory studies

The clinician should base the diagnostic evaluation on known or suspected contributing conditions. Obtain blood levels of any drugs and ensure that the patient has had a recent physical examination. The laboratory tests recommended for delirium may also be of value.

Differential diagnosis

If the typical precipitating events of an adjustment disorder are absent or indistinct, suspect drug toxicity, metabolic disturbance, cerebrovascular disease, early phase primary dementia, or delirium.

INTERPERSONAL INTERVENTION

The elderly patient taken to the ED by family members or caregivers should be given privacy. Obtain a history from the accompanying person (Minden, 1984). If the diagnosis is adjustment disorder, begin the interpersonal strategy, which takes the form of crisis intervention (Minden, 1984). Try to:

• help the patient discover a causal relationship between life events and onset of symptoms

• allow the patient to ventilate feelings without forcing him to do so

• convey empathy and respect for the patient

• remind the patient that his coping skills served him in the past

• impart a sense of purpose and optimism in reversing the emotional disorder.

The success of this strategy depends on the patient's premorbid personality, intellect, and current cognitive state. In all cases, the clinician can help the patient and family members by remaining optimistic. However, the immediate need for inpatient treatment takes precedence over crisis intervention in patients who are psychotic, grossly depressed, or suicidal.

PHARMACOLOGIC INTERVENTION

"Less is more" characterizes the drug treatment of adjustment problems in elderly patients (Walker and Covington, 1984). Because many psychotropic agents can impair cognitive function, deferring drug treatment is usually best. If the patient is already taking a psychotropic medication, the clinician must rule out drug toxicity as the cause of the problem. Adjustments in dosage can be considered later.

If psychotropic drugs must be prescribed, the dosage for an elderly person is one-third to one-half the usual adult dosage. Any side effects, such as orthostatic hypotension or sedation, are magnified in the elderly patient.

Do not initiate antidepressant therapy in the emergency setting. If necessary, a patient with mild anxiety, insomnia, or somatic complaints out of proportion to his condition can be given a small dose of a short-acting benzodiazepine. Appropriate drugs are alprazolam (Xanax) 0.25 mg, lorazepam (Ativan) 0.5 mg, or oxazepam (Serax) 10 mg up to three times daily.

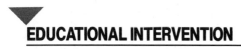

EDUCATIONAL INTERVENTION

Explain to the patient and family that adjustment disorders do not necessarily represent a serious illness or permanent deterioration and that the patient can probably return to his previous level of functioning. Suggest psychotherapy as a possible method of effecting the desired change in the patient's behavior, and emphasize the harmful effects of alcohol on the aging brain.

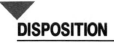

DISPOSITION

If an adjustment disorder appears to be a major depression or psychosis, the patient should be hospitalized. Suicide is the most serious potential consequence of failing to hospitalize a severely depressed or psychotic patient. If the patient is discharged, document any recommendations for antidepressant or other pharmacologic intervention, and notify the primary physician.

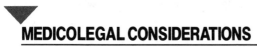

MEDICOLEGAL CONSIDERATIONS

Many elderly patients refuse treatment because they feel they have been forced to get help. Even if this feeling is justified, the clinician must choose between honoring the patient's refusal of treatment and addressing the family's demand for action. The key issue is patient competence. A competent patient has a right to refuse treatment. When the patient's health and safety are in jeopardy, however, the refusal can be temporarily overridden. The clinician can treat an incompetent patient but should try to obtain the family's consent first.

▼
IDENTIFYING THE PROBLEM: PSYCHOSIS

Psychotic symptoms in elderly patients can signal a life-threatening illness, so timely intervention is needed. The most common types of psychoses in the elderly population are delirium; organic delusional syndrome, usually with Alzheimer's disease; chronic mental illness, especially bipolar disorder; and major depression with psychotic features. The clinician can differentiate among psychotic disorders by reviewing the patient's history. For example, delirium has an acute onset, organic delusional syndrome develops gradually, chronic mental illness is obvious, and major depression is typically accompanied by apathy and suicidal ideation. In patients with bipolar disorder, mood swings accelerate in later life, although the episodes tend to be brief.

Mental status findings
The mental status findings in an elderly patient with delirium include clouded consciousness, disorientation, and hallucinations. A patient with organic delusional syndrome may be suspicious, have delusions of being poisoned or watched by others, and hide things and accuse others of stealing them. A bipolar disorder can cause such symptoms as irritability, grandiosity, poor social judgment, and decreased need for sleep. A patient suffering from major depression is apathetic, feels guilty and hopeless, and has suicidal thoughts and delusions of poverty or disease.

Physical findings
No specific physical findings aid in the diagnosis of a psychotic disorder. However, a long-standing episode of major depression can be accompanied by dehydration and malnutrition.

Laboratory studies
Beyond the investigation for causes of delirium and other organic conditions, further tests depend entirely on the clinician's judgment. In all cases, order tests for blood levels of any measurable medications.

Differential diagnosis

The main differential diagnosis is between functional psychosis and delirium. Make every effort to identify a reversible cause of the mental status changes; consider the possibility of prescription drug misuse, alcohol-related syndromes, and drug toxicity.

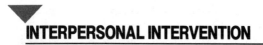

INTERPERSONAL INTERVENTION

A psychotic elderly patient may be suspicious, agitated, combative, or have a negative attitude. Emergency service staff members must be prepared to provide close, if not constant, supervision until the patient is treated or discharged. Encourage family members or friends to stay with the patient; their presence reassures the patient and reduces the likelihood that physical restraint will be needed.

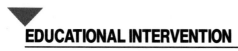

PHARMACOLOGIC INTERVENTION

Most psychotic elderly patients are admitted for inpatient treatment. If interim treatment is necessary, prescribe small doses of an antipsychotic agent. The use of rapid tranquilization in the elderly population has not been well studied. Therefore, a patient given single doses of a neuroleptic drug, such as haloperidol 0.25 to 1 mg I.M. or 0.5 to 1 mg orally, should be observed for at least 1 hour before the dose is repeated. Low-potency neuroleptic agents and benzodiazepines should be avoided in suspected cases of delirium.

EDUCATIONAL INTERVENTION

Direct all educational efforts toward the family. Inform them about the diagnosis, obtain their consent for treatment, and enlist their help in managing the patient.

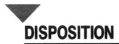

DISPOSITION

A newly psychotic patient should be treated in an inpatient setting. The clinician's time is better spent arranging the transfer rather than trying to reverse the psychosis in the emergency service. Symptoms in a chronically mentally ill person that were exacerbated by medication noncompliance may be treated now with the usual medications. If symptoms respond, discharge the patient. In these cases, give detailed instructions to the family members or caregiver and make plans for follow-up care.

MEDICOLEGAL CONSIDERATIONS

Because psychosis has variable effects on the elderly patient's ability to make treatment decisions, use the mental status examination to assess his competence. Be alert to the possibility that a patient is being forced into the hospital by family members. Any competent patient can refuse treatment. However, a psychotic patient who is a danger to himself or others or who cannot perform self-care may be subject to civil commitment.

REFERENCES

Diagnostic and Statistical Manual of Mental Disorders, 3rd ed., revised. Washington, D.C.: American Psychiatric Association, 1987.

Dubin, W.R., Weiss, K.J., and Dorn, J.M. "Pharmacotherapy of Psychiatric Emergencies," *Journal of Clinical Psychopharmacology* 6(4):210-222, August 1986.

Ellison, J., Hughes, D.H., and White, K.A. "An Emergency Psychiatry Update," *Hospital and Community Psychiatry* 40(3):250-260, March 1989.

Goodstein, R.K. "Common Clinical Problems in the Elderly Camouflaged by Ageism and Atypical Presentation," *Psychiatric Annals* 15(5):299-312, May 1985.

Hall, R.C.W., Feinsilver, D.L., and Holt, R.E. "Anticholinergic Psychosis: Differential Diagnosis and Management," *Psychosomatics* 22(7):581-587, July 1981.

Jenike, M.A. *Handbook of Geriatric Psychopharmacology.* Littleton, Mass.: PSG Publishing, 1985.

Minden, S.L. "Elderly Psychiatric Emergency Patients," in *Emergency Psychiatry: Concepts, Methods, and Practices.* Edited by Bassuk, E.L., and Birk, A.S. New York: Plenum Press, 1984.

Thompson, T.L. "Dementia," in *Textbook of Neuropsychiatry.* Edited by Hales, R.E., and Yudofsky, S.C. Washington, D.C.: American Psychiatric Press, 1987.

Walker, J.I., and Covington, T.R. "Psychiatric Disorders," in *Current Geriatric Therapy.* Edited by Covington, T.R., and Walker, J.I. Philadelphia: W.B. Saunders, 1984.

Wells, C.E. "Pseudodementia," *American Journal of Psychiatry* 136(7):895-900, July 1979.

15

DIFFICULT
SITUATIONS

A clinician working in the psychiatric emergency service has the difficult task of making quick decisions about strangers with major life disruptions. The types of patients described in previous chapters challenge one's diagnostic and therapeutic skills. Helping patients in crisis or reversing distressing drug side effects can be rewarding. At other times, however, frustration dominates, arising from a combination of the treatment setting, the patient's symptoms, and personal reactions to the patient (Hanke, 1984).

This chapter describes several troublesome clinical situations. Each clinician tends to develop a rapport with some patients and to struggle with others. Do not try to ignore negative reactions but rather use them as diagnostic clues about the patient (Hanke, 1984). Any clinician who experiences a negative reaction to a patient should leave the interview and confer with another staff member or supervisor. Use this opportunity to formulate a rational response, remembering that these feelings stem from the patient's problem. Keep in mind that a clinician can vent anger with other staff members; hostility directed toward the patient is always destructive and indicates a personal loss of control.

▼

IDENTIFYING THE PROBLEM: DRUG-SEEKING BEHAVIOR

Because medications are used to treat mental disorders, drug-seeking patients are naturally drawn to the psychiatric emergency setting. Drug-seeking behavior is seen in the addicted patient who fears withdrawal or is in acute withdrawal, the "recreational" drug user who comes to the emergency service seeking an economical and legal source of prescription drugs, and the "pseudopatient" who may want drugs to sell on the street. The clinician must distinguish between a patient in true withdrawal—a medical emergency—and one who is merely seeking drugs. Recognizing drug withdrawal is discussed in Chapter 5, Drug Abuse Emergencies.

Prescription drug abuse can be difficult to identify because patients do not necessarily share the same signs and symptoms. For example, a multidrug abuser—who mixes prescription drugs (usually sedatives, opioids, or stimulants) with street drugs and alcohol—has various complaints, including anxiety, depression, insomnia, and pain. The plausibility of these complaints varies with the sophistication of the patient. Because the diagnosis of most psychiatric disorders largely depends on what the patient says, the prescription drug abuser takes advantage of established procedures. A patient who abuses prescription drugs may report, "I lost my prescription" or "I can't get in touch with my doctor." Learn to recognize the typical features of abuse; then rely on intuition and experience to diagnose prescription drug abuse.

Mental status findings

Expect unusual or incredible complaints of anxiety or depression, intolerance of the interview and laboratory tests, refusal of nondrug interventions, use of various pressure tactics, and early requests for a specific medication.

Physical findings

Look for a history of trauma (such as fractures and burns) not explained by the patient's occupation, skin infections, hepatitis, heart valve infections, seizures, pulmonary disorders suggesting cocaine freebasing, or general debilitation (Wilford, 1981).

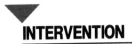

INTERVENTION

The immediate task is to determine whether an emergency exists and, if not, whether the request for drugs is reasonable and appropriate. Being alert to prescription drug abuse does not mean turning away patients who may simply have run out of medication.

The patient's history reveals the course of the illness and the current treatment. In the absence of a medical emergency, contact the prescribing physician to verify the legitimacy of the patient's request. Asking the patient to wait for the results of the evaluation also reveals his motivation: the typical multidrug abuser is not likely to stay, whereas the patient with nothing to hide will remain.

DISPOSITION

For patients specifically seeking prescription drugs, identify legitimate cases by contacting the prescribing physician or by checking hospital records. "Well-known" patients are usually recognized by staff members as habitual drug seekers, but be careful not to dismiss such persons before excluding true drug withdrawal. Antisocial, malingering, and multidrug-abusing persons usually make their own disposition by exiting the emergency service, sometimes making threatening or insulting remarks on the way out.

For the suspected drug abuser who stays, consider these options:
• Tell the patient that no emergency exists, and refer him to an outpatient setting. Do not be intimidated by the patient; be assertive without being hostile.
• Notify hospital security if the patient becomes threatening or appears on the verge of losing control.
• If the patient seems to be making a legitimate request, consider prescribing antianxiety or hypnotic benzodiazepines, but limit the supply to 1 to 3 days.
• Give the patient a courteous but firm message that prescriptions are best handled by his primary care physician, and volunteer to notify the physician.

▼

IDENTIFYING THE PROBLEM: ACQUIRED IMMUNODEFICIENCY SYNDROME

Psychiatric emergency clinicians are increasingly called on to evaluate and treat known or suspected cases of acquired immunodeficiency syndrome (AIDS), an infectious disease (Kelen et al., 1989; Ellison et al., 1989; Perry, 1990). Staff members may fear contact with those infected with the human immunodeficiency virus (HIV) or those with AIDS. Clinicians may resist working with "hopeless" patients. Furthermore, clinicians and staff members may have negative attitudes toward persons believed to be predisposed to AIDS, such as homosexuals and drug abusers.

An AIDS patient may display neuropsychiatric manifestations of HIV infection—anxiety, depression, psychosis, dementia, and delirium. In other cases, the patient may be anxious or depressed because of the diagnosis of AIDS, the stress of chronic illness, impoverishment, social stigma, or anticipation of death. AIDS patients may also come to the emergency service for treatment of depression and grief after the deaths of friends who also had AIDS.

Public hysteria caused by the AIDS epidemic has increased the number of nonaffected patients who are excessively concerned about contracting the disease (Ellison et al., 1989). Delusional and obsessive patients make demands for testing and do not respond to reassurance.

Autopsy studies show an 80% incidence of neuropathological findings among adult victims of AIDS. Approximately half of these patients had clinically apparent neurologic disorders before death (Dalakas et al., 1989). The following HIV-related central nervous system (CNS) diseases may be initially diagnosed during a psychiatric emergency visit: aseptic meningitis; vacuolar myelopathy; progressive or static HIV encephalopathy of childhood; AIDS dementia complex; opportunistic viral infections; progressive multifocal leukoencephalopathy; herpes simplex and zoster; cytomegalovirus; opportunistic nonviral infections; toxoplasma, cryptococcus, *Candida*, coccidioides, *Aspergillus*, and other fungal infections; *Mycobacterium tuberculosis, M. avium*, or *M. intracellulare* infections; *Listeria* and *Nocardia* infections; and primary CNS lymphomas (Dalakas et al., 1989).

▼
INTERVENTIONS

Every clinician has a duty to treat persons in distress, including those with AIDS. Include AIDS as part of the differential diagnosis of all organic and functional mental disorders. Because a neuropsychiatric presentation of AIDS may be the first clinical manifestation of the disease, a timely diagnosis can have a significant impact on the patient's health and the welfare of others. Thus, be informed about treatment resources and referral networks in the community.

To prepare for psychiatric treatment of a known or suspected AIDS patient, a clinician should:

• consider HIV infection when evaluating a broad range of psychiatric complaints

• determine the patient's drug use and sexual habits, known exposure to HIV, and current preventive practices

• identify and modify staff members' negative attitudes through education

• reduce staff members' fears of contracting AIDS from patients through education

• maintain procedures for the proper disposal of needles and bodily fluids of AIDS patients (Ellison et al., 1989; Kelen et al., 1989).

Crisis intervention techniques are most appropriate in treating the AIDS patient with an adjustment disorder. These techniques include identifying the source of the distress, reviewing the patient's coping skills, mobilizing a support system, and developing an interim plan for follow-up care. When the adjustment disorder is complicated by drug or alcohol abuse or suicidal ideation, the patient should be hospitalized. Be aware of social networks dedicated to helping AIDS patients with medical and legal problems, and contact these services immediately as part of the intervention.

The AIDS patient without a preexisting psychosis can have a delusional disorder, hallucinations, or delirium. The principal diagnostic consideration is HIV-induced organic disorder. Other considerations are drug side effects, intoxication, infections, and reactive psychosis (breakdown under the stress of the illness). Because psychosis, especially delirium, may imply a deterioration of the patient's overall condition, contact his primary care physician. Most patients with psychotic symptoms should be hospitalized. If the psychotic patient must be tranquilized, consider administering a high-potency neuroleptic agent, such as haloperidol (Haldol) 5 to 10 mg orally or 5 mg I.M.

Some patients who are not at risk for HIV infection have a delusional or obsessive preoccupation with the disease. In such cases, take the usual history of risk and exposure factors, and do not dismiss the patient's fears before ruling out all risk factors. Do not offer AIDS testing on demand, unless authorized by a medical specialist. Without a medical basis for the patient's concern, focus on treating the patient's psychiatric illness, particularly the reasons for the preoccupation with AIDS.

▼
MEDICOLEGAL CONSIDERATIONS

Mandatory reporting of AIDS cases to public health officials is imminent (Nissenbaum, 1989). Under such laws, clinicians would be required to report all cases of AIDS but would be protected from breach of confidentiality. Whether these laws would protect clinicians who warn potential sexual contacts without the patient's consent is unclear. Emergency service staff members should be aware of the local reporting requirements, and a written policy and procedure should be in place. Until the law is established, act to protect potential victims of an AIDS patient who is determined to infect others. Voluntary hospitalization or civil commitment can be used in these situations. Whether calling the police constitutes a breach of confidentiality depends on the seriousness and imminence of the threat as well as the state's statutes and case law.

Assess the AIDS patient with dementia or delirium for clinical competency, especially before making treatment decisions.

▼
IDENTIFYING THE PROBLEM: CONVERSION DISORDER (CONVERSION HYSTERIA)

Patients with conversion disorder experience a loss of or alteration in physical functioning that suggests a physical disorder. A psychosocial stressor usually precedes onset of symptoms—a man who is humiliated in business becomes sexually dysfunctional, a woman who finds out her husband is unfaithful becomes blind, a man enraged at an authority figure has arm paralysis, a woman with an urge to run away develops foot anesthesia. The person does not intentionally produce the symptom, as in malingering. The symptom is not a culturally sanctioned response pattern, and, after appropriate investigation, cannot be explained by a known physical disorder. Physical symptoms can be suspiciously strange, and their distribution does not conform to anatomy. A common example is "stocking" paralysis or anesthesia (a deficit in the shape of a sock), which does not conform to either central or peripheral nerve pathways. Persons with conversion disorder are not phony or crazy. Symptoms are an expression of emotional conflict and should be treated seriously.

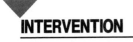

INTERVENTION

Although dramatic and upsetting to persons around the patient, conversion disorder is highly treatable in the emergency setting. The patient is usually accompanied by the person with whom he is in conflict. Separate the patient from the accompanying person, and obtain a history from each party in separate interviews.

If thorough physical and neurologic examinations confirm that the patient does not have an organic condition, provide a simple psychodynamic formulation of the problem; for example, "You were so angry you could kill" or "Your feelings were so strong you couldn't move." The experience of being understood usually helps the patient to recover function; if not, do not force the patient to give up the symptoms, but refer him for outpatient psychotherapy (Walker, 1983).

A pharmacologic approach can also be effective, using the amobarbital (Amytal) interview described in Chapter 6, Schizophrenia and Mania. The goal is a rapid dissolution of the patient's defenses and a return to baseline functioning. The amobarbital interview does not replace the need for subsequent psychotherapy, however.

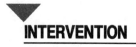

IDENTIFYING THE PROBLEM: HYPOCHONDRIASIS

Hypochondriasis is characterized by a preoccupation with and fear of having a serious disease, based on the patient's interpretation of physical signs or sensations as evidence of physical illness. Such patients are ubiquitous in the medical community and are sometimes pejoratively labeled, shunned, or mismanaged.

Suspect hypochondriasis when an appropriate physical evaluation does not support the diagnosis of any physical disorder that can account for the patient's signs or symptoms. A hypochondriacal patient does not respond to medical reassurance. As with other somatoform disorders, the patient is not psychotic or delusional.

INTERVENTION

Do not spend time on extensive diagnostic testing of the patient, and avoid hostile confrontations because the patient will leave to go "doctor shopping." The best approach is to maintain an understanding attitude without reinforcing the patient's behavior.

IDENTIFYING THE PROBLEM: SOMATIZATION DISORDER (BRIQUET'S SYNDROME)

A patient with somatization disorder has a history of many physical complaints or a belief that he is sickly; the disorder begins before age 30 and persists for several years. The patient describes at least 13 physical complaints. Typical symptoms are vomiting (other than during pregnancy), pain in extremities, shortness of breath when at rest, amnesia, difficulty swallowing, burning sensation in the sexual organs or rectum (other than during intercourse), and painful menstruation.

These symptoms are considered evidence of somatization disorder if no organic pathology or pathophysiological mechanism accounts for the complaint. In addition, when real disease exists, the resulting social or occupational impairment is grossly in excess of what is expected. The patient's complaints do not occur only during an acute anxiety attack, and symptoms cause the patient to take medication, see a physician, or alter his life-style.

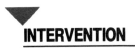

INTERVENTION

Insist that the patient establish or maintain an ongoing relationship with a psychotherapist, and repeat this message as necessary, because such patients usually return to the emergency service. To decrease the intensity of complaints, be available to listen to the patient and to mediate between him and medical-surgical specialists who may have been consulted about the original complaint. The main risk to the patient is unnecessary medical procedures.

MEDICOLEGAL CONSIDERATIONS

Suspect malingering when the patient willfully describes or exaggerates symptoms for an external (usually monetary) gain. Personal injury litigation is the most prevalent form of somatoform malingering. The patient, who may have been injured in the past, attempts to raise the amount of a settlement or award by perpetuating physical complaints. In the psychiatric emergency setting, such a patient might request "documentation" of a pain problem. Upon questioning, the patient may admit that he was sent by an attorney. Refer such requests to an appropriate outpatient setting, such as a pain clinic.

Also be careful not to diagnose somatization disorder prematurely, thereby failing to identify an organic condition. Even if the patient is well known, treat each complaint with enough interest to avoid a charge of negligence.

IDENTIFYING THE PROBLEM: FACTITIOUS DISORDER (MUNCHAUSEN SYNDROME)

The patient with factitious disorder intentionally produces physical or psychological symptoms and has a psychological need to assume the sick role, as evidenced by an absence of external incentives for the behavior, such as economic gain, better care, or physical well-being. This lack of ulterior motives distinguishes factitious disorder from malingering. The syndrome occurs independent of another disorder, such as schizophrenia.

Patients with factitious disorder commonly seek treatment in general hospitals and emergency departments (EDs) after going to great lengths to induce illness; they may mutilate, poison, or otherwise harm themselves and, to prolong illness, may intentionally underdose or overdose with medications or undo the work of physicians (for instance, by rubbing dirt in wounds or pulling out intravenous lines). Suspect factitious disorder in patients who are accident-prone or slow to heal.

The typical patient has a dramatic clinical presentation, is a pathological liar, argues with hospital personnel, has extensive medical knowledge, and demands pain medication. The patient's history reveals evidence of multiple surgical procedures and extensive traveling to seek treatment (Walker, 1983).

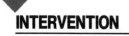

INTERVENTION

A patient with factitious disorder has a mental disorder. Although the patient's psychological need to be sick may respond to treatment, he can engender frustration, even rage, among clinicians, especially if they feel duped. Gently confront the patient with the diagnosis. If discussing the patient's need to be sick is not effective, a psychiatric consultation and outpatient psychotherapy are indicated. Consider hospitalizing the patient only if real symptoms, such as psychosis, appear.

MEDICOLEGAL CONSIDERATIONS

A patient who contributes to his own illness, fabricates stories, and manipulates medical professionals is likely to develop a reputation as an undesirable person. Thus, resist temptations to disregard the patient's complaints, which could lead to misdiagnosis. Although the patient lies about his health, he does have real physical injuries, albeit self-inflicted, and the clinician who overlooks a genuine problem may be judged negligent.

Because the patient has a psychiatric disorder, plan to control his self-destructive impulses. For example, injecting oneself with insulin and seeking attention for hypoglycemia could be construed as "imminent danger to self," which satisfies civil commitment standards. Most patients are not committed, however, either because they need nonpsychiatric treatment or because they volunteer for psychiatric hospitalization.

▼ IDENTIFYING THE PROBLEM: MALINGERING

Malingering is the intentional production of false or grossly exaggerated physical or psychological symptoms for ulterior motives, such as avoiding military conscription or service, dodging work, acquiring financial compensation, evading criminal prosecution, obtaining drugs, or securing better living conditions. Suspect malingering if the patient is referred by an attorney or has a lawsuit pending, if a marked discrepancy exists between the person's claimed stress or disability and the objective findings, if the patient refuses to cooperate with the assessment or treatment, or if the patient has an antisocial personality.

Malingering is not a mental disorder. In contrast to patients with factitious disorder, the malingerer's goal is not to maintain the sick role but to achieve some external gain. Malingering patients can be distinguished from those with somatoform disorders by their willfulness and apparent absence of emotional conflict in relation to their symptoms. Once the clinician "unmasks" a malingerer, the patient usually disappears from treatment and repeats the behavior elsewhere.

Several types of malingerers are commonly seen in the psychiatric emergency setting. Prescription drug abusers recite symptoms or act out a caricature of a mental disorder to obtain drugs, such as benzodiazepines or barbiturates. Others arrive with "documentation" of a disorder—attention deficit disorder, narcolepsy, depression—to obtain stimulants. This type of malingering is commonly associated with antisocial personality disorder. The clinician should examine suspected prescription drug abusers and ask them to wait before taking further action.

Many deinstitutionalized patients live on the streets in good weather and try to gain admission into mental hospitals (for "three hots and a cot") at other times. Although these persons have real illnesses, their exaggeration or fabrication of symptoms is a conscious effort to secure better living conditions. Many patients are so adept at finding a way into hospitals that they arrive at the ED ready for a trip ("the suitcase sign").

Occasionally, a person comes to the emergency service and requests a note to an employer, probation officer, or creditor. The goal is to have the clinician validate a mental problem as an excuse for delinquent behavior. Other persons may seek documentation of a mental problem to obtain public assistance or other government entitlements.

The emergency services clinician may encounter a person with atypical complaints who has had an automobile or industrial accident. Even if the clinician has no reason to suspect malingering at the outset, the patient's lack of real distress and the connection with litigation should prompt further questioning. The malingerer's purpose is to build a legal case on documentation of a fabricated illness.

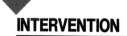

INTERVENTION

The primary strategy for dealing with the malingerer is to avoid struggles and verbally aggressive exchanges. Avoid the temptation to punish the patient. The best course of action is to explain that the patient's complaint does not require the requested treatment. Explain and document the reason for denying any patient requests for medication or documentation.

Many deinstitutionalized patients are clever enough to escalate the situation. For example, some patients have memorized the language of the civil commitment law and state, "I am dangerous to myself and others." Such cases fall between malingering and factitious disorder. If the patient's judgment is sufficiently impaired to put him at real risk, consider hospitalizing him. Refer other patients to an appropriate inpatient setting, a shelter, or an outpatient or day hospitalization service.

MEDICOLEGAL CONSIDERATIONS

Be careful not to prematurely diagnose a patient as a malingerer; overlooking a disorder could have serious complications. For example, refusing a chronic patient who seeks shelter might motivate the patient to cause actual harm to himself or others to impress the clinician. Although the clinician might have no legal duty to control the patient's actions, a negative outcome could result in a lawsuit.

IDENTIFYING THE PROBLEM: HOMELESSNESS

Many of the urban homeless are both severely impoverished and chronically mentally ill. Psychiatric emergency services and social services personnel are frequently called on to work with homeless persons after their immediate physical problems (thermal injuries, infections, congestive heart failure, trauma) are treated. Although the typical "street person" is difficult to characterize, such persons are likely to suffer from one or more psychiatric illnesses, including schizophrenia, alcoholism, drug abuse, organic mental disorders, and personality disorders. Because of the number of biopsychosocial pathologies seen in street people, many resources must be devoted to their treatment (Ellison et al., 1989).

A clinician may have difficulty communicating with the street person. Other staff members seem to have a better rapport with these patients and can best assess their needs. If possible, staff members should serve as liaisons between the patient and the clinician. The clinician's initial task is to determine what the patient wants (shelter, medical attention, neuroleptic medication). Since many patients are brought in by police, the chief complaint may be obscure.

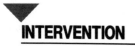

INTERVENTION

Helping the patient to clean up and offering food and drink may be the best ways to engage the patient and learn about him — if he is schizophrenic or has stopped taking antipsychotic medication, for example. With such details, consider restarting the medication; however, encourage the patient to enter a day treatment program. Some street people may be demented because of head trauma or nutritional deficiencies. If possible, these patients should be hospitalized for further evaluation. As a general rule, screen all street persons for medical illnesses. The importance of careful evaluation is illustrated by the case of the "typical street person" who actually had severe hypothyroidism (Shader and Greenblatt, 1987).

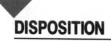

DISPOSITION

In contrast to the impoverished patient, the mentally ill homeless person is commonly resistant to a meaningful change in life-style. A caring, nonthreatening clinician may be able to place the patient into the mental health care system. Walking the patient to a drop-in center or day hospital may be worthwhile.

MEDICOLEGAL CONSIDERATIONS

That homeless mentally ill persons choose to live on the street may seem incomprehensible, yet many do so consciously even though the choice is associated with a psychotic illness. When street persons come to the psychiatric emergency service, they are not asking the clinician to run their lives. Therefore, unless the patient is incompetent or dangerous, the clinician usually must honor the patient's refusal of neuroleptic medication or medical care. Overly aggressive treatment infringes on the patient's privacy.

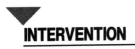

IDENTIFYING THE PROBLEM: TELEPHONE CALLERS

Most emergency services have hotlines to answer telephone calls for help, advice, or crisis intervention. The clinician has a duty to respond, but with the limitations imposed by the situation: no face-to-face contact, physical control, or visual confirmation of what the caller states. The clinician answering telephone calls should be prepared for many different situations (Fauman and Fauman, 1981).

INTERVENTION

First, ask the caller to give his name, address, phone number, and any details of recent clinical contacts. Since many callers refuse to provide this information, inquire about the reason for the secrecy but do not threaten negative consequences if the patient refuses to answer.

For routine psychiatric or drug side effect questions, provide a direct answer and remind the patient that a personal visit may be necessary. If the patient threatens suicide or claims to have taken an overdose of drugs, remember that he is asking for help and does not want to die. If the patient is serious about accepting help, he will give identifying information. Also obtain details of the type and amount of substances ingested (Gilmore, 1984). Then end the conversation and contact family members, friends, neighbors, police, rescue squads, or other resources that can help the patient (Fauman and Fauman, 1981).

Be careful to maintain control when speaking with nuisance callers—individuals who intentionally abuse crisis hotlines. The best approach is to inform the caller that the hotline is for persons who want help and direction to an appropriate resource for a legitimate problem. Also tell the caller that tying up the line deprives others of needed attention.

Do not honor a caller's request for prescriptions. Fulfilling such a request is a serious ethical error that could lead to a liability claim.

▼

IDENTIFYING THE PROBLEM: BORDERLINE PERSONALITY DISORDER

Patients with borderline personality disorder invariably induce negative reactions in hospital staff. These patients, many of whom are women, have some or all of the following symptoms: unstable and intense relationships, impulsivity (sex, gambling, drugs, self-abuse), marked mood shifts, disturbed sense of self, inappropriate and intense anger, suicidal behavior or threats, feelings of emptiness or boredom, and panic over real or imagined abandonment (*DSM-III-R*, 1987; Groves, 1987).

Borderline patients have diverse complaints. In some cases, the presenting complaint may be psychosis, with or without complicating substance abuse. The differential diagnosis is broad, since these patients "border" on several areas of psychopathology. Their rage at staff members, rejection of help, and spiteful threats make them difficult to treat. Repeat patients may have sensitized the staff to dread them. To a degree, the diagnosis of borderline personality is more stigmatizing than that of schizophrenia (Hanke, 1984).

▼

INTERPERSONAL INTERVENTION

Managing the borderline patient is also an exercise in managing one's own feelings; the manipulation and rage coming from the patient are formidable barriers to interaction. The clinician must not take the patient's behavior personally. These patients usually hate themselves and spread this hate by accusing others of mistreatment. The clinician must remember that the patient's rage is a function of the psychopathology, not necessarily a valid criticism of the treatment.

An effective interpersonal intervention begins by setting limits (Hanke, 1984), which means spelling out the rules: Patients must not hurt themselves or throw things, and they must put their feelings into words. As with the violent patient, many borderline patients on the verge of losing control are more secure when given specific, but not punitive, guidelines. Departures from the rules must be constantly brought to the patient's attention to break through impasses in the intervention. The patient's usual problems with other persons are repeated with the clinician. Pointing this out is an important part of the learning process for the borderline patient and can be accomplished in the emergency setting.

Sometimes another staff member is more successful with a particular patient, making a team approach feasible. Staff members must maintain effective communication among themselves because the borderline patient can set one staff member against another. When necessary, call the patient's therapist (consent may not be needed in an emergency but should be obtained if possibie), who can provide missing pieces of the patient's history and advice on the intervention approach. The patient may be in crisis because of stress produced during a therapy session. Although the patient may complain bitterly that the therapist is worthless, he is usually reassured to know that the therapist was contacted.

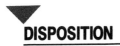

PHARMACOLOGIC INTERVENTION

For a patient experiencing psychotic episodes, the clinician can administer a low dose of a neuroleptic agent, such as haloperidol 1 to 2 mg or thioridazine (Mellaril) 50 to 100 mg orally. A nonpsychotic but panicked patient can be given a benzodiazepine, such as lorazepam (Ativan) 1 to 2 mg, unless the patient is a known substance abuser.

DISPOSITION

Plan to return the borderline patient in crisis to his therapist for a more thorough resolution. This disposition can be complicated because the crisis may be precipitated by the therapy itself, especially the patient's feelings about the therapist (transference). The clinician should briefly hospitalize the patient (with the therapist's knowledge) only when the patient exhibits psychotic or self-destructive symptoms. Refer to a therapist any borderline patient who is not in regular treatment.

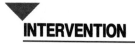

IDENTIFYING THE PROBLEM: ANTISOCIAL PERSONALITY DISORDER

Patients with antisocial personality disorder are rarely in genuine distress but use the emergency service for some other purpose, such as obtaining drugs or avoiding criminal prosecution. Sometimes these patients are prescription drug abusers. Antisocial persons may violate the rights of others, lie, or break the law and feel no remorse. They are typically brought in by the police for disruptive behavior and proceed to create fear and hatred among staff members.

INTERVENTION

Address the patient's chief complaint without yielding to unreasonable demands for drugs or services. If the patient is intoxicated or violent and has been brought in by the police, ask them to stay until the patient is under control. If the patient entered the emergency service alone, call hospital security at the first sign of threatening or disruptive behavior. (Management of violent patients is described in Chapter 7, Violent Behavior.) The interpersonal intervention is similar to that for the borderline patient. Use a direct, confrontational approach to the patient's lying and manipulativeness (Hanke, 1984).

MEDICOLEGAL CONSIDERATIONS

Although patients with personality disorder appear dysfunctional, they are rarely psychotic or clinically incompetent. Therefore, assume that they are able to make decisions about their health care. In addition, such patients retain the right to refuse treatment, unless they are demonstrably dangerous. Any use of restraints or involuntary medication must be well documented.

The criteria for commitment are functional, not based on a diagnosis. Persons with borderline, antisocial, or other personality disorders may have homicidal or suicidal tendencies, thereby fulfilling the commitment criteria. Document the patient's behavior in detail. In addition to noting any personality problems, make a primary diagnosis of adjustment disorder, depression, or brief psychosis. In this way, the commitment is clearly based on an illness rather than simply a maladaptive behavior pattern.

A clinician who treats patients with personality disorders can become the target of a lawsuit. Some patients act out of rage against a perceived wrong by the clinician; others make a sport of suing professionals. Liability problems can also arise if the clinician acts on sadistic feelings toward the patient or engages in sexual relations with the patient.

▼

IDENTIFYING THE PROBLEM: LANGUAGE BARRIERS

Medical centers in general and psychiatric emergency services in particular care for many patients who do not speak English. In ethnic neighborhoods or those with immigrant populations, the best approach is to have at least one bilingual staff member on duty each day. A general hospital usually has a bilingual person available for help in a crisis. When such assistance is unavailable, use a phrase book to help assess a patient's chief complaint and the urgency of the situation. Interpreter resources should be part of the emergency service's resource manual. Local ethnic churches may be a reliable source of interpreters.

▼

IDENTIFYING THE PROBLEM: THE DEVELOPMENTALLY DISABLED PATIENT

Because the number of deinstitutionalized developmentally disabled (mentally retarded or brain-injured) citizens living in the community is increasing, emergency services can expect to see more patients referred from community living centers. Adjustment disorders and uncontrolled or self-destructive behavior are the most common problems seen in developmentally disabled persons. Except with the mildly retarded person, the clinician may have difficulty obtaining a coherent history and valid mental status examination.

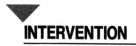

INTERVENTION

Do not ignore the patient, and encourage family members and friends to stay with him at all times. The parent or caregiver can serve as an interpreter of the patient's language and nonverbal behavior. Do not make a diagnosis of psychosis too quickly; a developmentally disabled patient may appear regressed when suffering from an adjustment disorder. In most cases, an easily identifiable external stressor — a change in staffing at the community residence, roommate problems, or visits from relatives — breaks adaptive behavior. Even if the stressor is identified, investigate whether seizures or other medical conditions are contributing to the problem and whether the patient usually takes psychotropic medications. Give the patient a simplified but direct interpretation of the problem, and reinforce his ability to cope with the situation. Keep pharmacologic intervention to a minimum, and make every effort to return the patient to his usual living arrangements.

IDENTIFYING THE PROBLEM: DISPOSITION DIFFICULTIES

Many chronically mentally ill patients are difficult to place in hospitals or residential settings. These patients may be psychotic or have a disagreeable personality or history of noncompliance. A patient who has no medical insurance is also hard to place. Such patients can remain in crisis centers for days. With appropriate emergency treatment, the patient's problem may resolve and symptoms may recede, allowing for an outpatient disposition.

To avoid having to care for a chronically ill patient indefinitely, each emergency service should have a resource manual that lists local and remote hospitals (both general and psychiatric), adult shelters, and specialized services (such as Veterans Administration services). In addition, one or more staff members should have a friendly liaison relationship with the community mental health in-patient unit to facilitate admission later.

Sometimes, a patient is dropped off at the crisis center by family members or boarding home personnel with the message "He's yours!" This situation may be the culmination of long-standing do-mestic strife or a mismatch at a community residence. The patient is usually chronically psychotic or elderly and demented.

In this situation, keep the third party involved and avoid giving the impression that he is relieved of responsibility by having brought the patient to the emergency service. If the crisis is acute, hospitalize the patient. When hospitalization is not indicated, the disposition can become complicated. If the clinician cannot resolve the inter-personal problem between the patient and the caregiver, either by mediating the dispute or by medicating the patient so that the caregiver can manage him, an alternative placement may be the only solution.

Effective communication with social service agencies is critical. If the patient is clinically competent, he should participate in the decision making. If the patient is incompetent, the clinician should attempt to locate responsible relatives who can assist in disposition planning. If domestic or institutional abuse is suspected, local re-porting requirements may mandate the involvement of a protective agency.

REFERENCES

Dalakas, M., et al. "AIDS and the Nervous System," *JAMA* 261(16):2396-2399, April 28, 1989.

Diagnostic and Statistical Manual of Mental Disorders, 3rd ed., revised. Wash-ington, D.C. American Psychiatric Association, 1987.

Ellison, J.M., Hughes, D.H., and White, K.A. "An Emergency Psychiatry Update," *Hospital and Community Psychiatry* 40(3):250-260, March 1989.

Fauman, B.J., and Fauman, M.A. *Emergency Psychiatry for the House Officer.* Baltimore: Williams and Wilkins, 1981.

Gilmore, B.S. "The Telephone in Psychiatric Emergencies," in *Emergency Psy-chiatry: Concepts, Methods, and Practices.* Edited by Bassuk, E.L., and Birk, A.W. New York: Plenum Press, 1984.

Groves, J.E. "Borderline Patients," in *Massachusetts General Hospital Hand-book of General Hospital Psychiatry.* Edited by Hackett, T., and Cassem, E. Lit-tleton, Mass.: PSG Publishing, 1987.

Hanke, N. *Handbook of Emergency Psychiatry.* Lexington, Mass.: Collamore Press, 1984.

Kelen, G.D., et al. "Human Immunodeficiency Virus Infection in Emergency Department Patients," *JAMA* 262(4):516-522, July 28, 1989.

Nissenbaum, G.D. "A Physician's Duty to Disclose That His Patient Has AIDS," *New Jersey Medicine* 86(2):123-125, February 1989.

Perry, S.W. "Organic Mental Disorders Caused by HIV: Update on Early Diagnosis and Treatment," *American Journal of Psychiatry* 147:696-710, 1990.

Shader, R.I., and Greenblatt, D.J. "Back to Basics — Diagnosis Before Treatment: Homelessness, Hypothyroidism, Aging, and Lithium," *Journal of Clinical Psychopharmacology* 7(6):375-376, December 1987.

Walker, J.I. *Psychiatric Emergencies: Intervention and Resolution.* Philadelphia: J.B. Lippincott, 1983.

Wilford, B.B. *Drug Abuse: A Guide for the Primary Care Physician.* Chicago: American Medical Association, 1981.

16

PSYCHOTROPIC DRUG REACTIONS

The widespread use of psychotropic medications has caused many patients to seek help because of drug toxicity. In such cases, the emergency clinician's goals include rapidly reversing the toxicity, counseling and educating the patient on how to prevent further problems, and encouraging him to pursue follow-up care with the prescribing physician or clinic.

GENERAL CONSIDERATIONS

Because patients seen in the emergency service for drug reactions are being treated elsewhere, the clinician has a dual role: to treat the patient and to preserve the continuity of the therapy. Perhaps the most important clinical responsibility in this area is alertness to psychotropic drug side effects, especially in vulnerable populations such as elderly patients.

In general, the clinician should take the following approach to patients with psychotropic drug toxicity:

• Verify which drugs the patient is taking by having the patient bring in the medication, asking a family member or caregiver, calling the prescribing physician or clinic, or ordering a blood or urine drug screen.

• Ask the patient how the medication is taken, especially whether the patient is ingesting more than the prescribed amount without telling the primary care physician.

• Treat the drug toxicity but leave the overall treatment strategy to the prescribing physician.

• Suspect prescription drug abuse in patients who repeatedly ask for controlled substances or appear to be fabricating side effects.

• Educate the patient about the problem, suggest that the patient discuss it with his physician, and tell him how to avoid future problems.

• Inform the prescribing physician of the contact with the patient, especially if a change in medication is indicated.

▼
ANTIPSYCHOTICS (NEUROLEPTICS)

Chronically psychotic persons living in community residences are commonly treated with high doses of a high-potency oral or long-acting intramuscular (depot) neuroleptic (antipsychotic) agent. Because the patient's clinic appointments may be 2 to 4 weeks apart, the clinician in the psychiatric emergency service or hospital may be the one to discover and treat drug side effects. The side effects of antipsychotic agents are so numerous that the interested reader should consult a textbook of psychopharmacology (Baldessarini, 1985; Mason and Granacher, 1980). Fortunately, most drug reactions are not emergencies, and many patients can be referred to their treating physicians.

General effects

Antipsychotic drugs have specific effects on dopamine systems and general effects on alertness. Common central nervous system (CNS) effects caused by these agents are sedation (drowsiness or "drugged" feeling), ataxia (unsteady gait or incoordination), slurred speech, dysphoria (generalized emotional discomfort), and loss of energy or initiative.

Differential diagnosis. For psychotic patients receiving antipsychotic drugs, the differential diagnosis for drug side effects includes primary symptoms of schizophrenia (apathy, dysphoria), interaction with alcohol or another sedative or hypnotic agent, depression, and metabolic or traumatic brain dysfunction.

Interpersonal intervention. After the differential diagnoses are ruled out, the clinician should advise the patient to discontinue the medication for the rest of the day and to contact the prescribing physician as soon as possible. The patient should be told not to engage in activities in which sedation would be hazardous – for example, driving a car.

Educational intervention. Before the patient leaves the emergency service, the clinician should explain that the side effects indicate that the drug is working, but that adjustments in dosage may be needed. For a patient recently placed on an antipsychotic agent, the clinician can point out that the sedation should be temporary. For other patients, such as those recently discharged from an acute care hospital on high doses of medication, the clinician can begin to educate them about the difference between acute and maintenance doses and suggest that they continue this discussion with the prescribing physician.

Neurologic effects

Neuroleptic drugs act diffusely on dopamine receptors in the brain, producing both antipsychotic effects and unwanted motor effects, or extrapyramidal symptoms (EPS). As a rule, the more potent the neuroleptic drug, the higher the risk for EPS, although any neuroleptic agent can cause EPS.

Extrapyramidal symptoms

The clinician should be familiar with the emergency treatment of EPS.

Akinesia. This syndrome, marked by a loss of spontaneous movement, is related to parkinsonism and may occur in conjunction with it. The patient is drowsy and looks and acts "washed out." Muscle rigidity, cogwheeling (a ratchetlike feeling when limbs are passively moved), and tremor are typically present (Mason and Granacher, 1980). Akinesia can progress to a catatonic-like state, which must be differentiated from catatonia itself and from neuroleptic malignant syndrome.

Because akinesia results from dopamine blockade, the drug of choice is an antiparkinsonian agent, such as diphenhydramine (Benadryl) 50 mg or benztropine (Cogentin) 2 mg, I.M. or I.V. The akinetic patient usually responds in several minutes to 1 hour. If no response occurs, the clinician can repeat the dose once. If successful, the drug should be continued orally (25 mg of diphenhydramine two to four times daily or 1 mg of benztropine twice daily).

Bear in mind that antiparkinsonian drugs are not benign and have serious toxic effects of their own, including delirium (central anticholinergic syndrome), euphoria or dysphoria, urine retention, glaucoma exacerbation, constipation, dry mouth, blurred vision, diminished sweating (possibly hyperthermia), and tachycardia. These effects are more severe in elderly patients and in those taking low-potency neuroleptic drugs.

An alternative initial intervention is to switch the akinetic patient from a high-potency to a low-potency antipsychotic agent, such as chlorpromazine (Thorazine) or thioridazine (Mellaril).

Parkinsonism. Sometimes called pseudoparkinsonism because it mimics Parkinson's disease, this syndrome is the most common EPS (Mason and Granacher, 1980). Key physical findings in patients with parkinsonism are shuffling or unsteady gait; resting tremor, usually of the "pillrolling" type; loss of expressive movements or masklike face; muscle rigidity; and drooling.

Elderly patients are especially susceptible to drug-induced parkinsonism. The clinician can distinguish parkinsonism from Parkinson's disease because the drug effect occurs after the introduction of the drug, whereas the disease has an insidious onset.

Like akinesia, this syndrome is readily reversed by antiparkinsonian drugs of the anticholinergic or antihistaminic type, such as diphenhydramine, benztropine, and trihexyphenidyl (Artane). The dopamine agonist drugs, such as levodopa-carbidopa (Sinemet), that are used to treat Parkinson's disease should not be used for drug-induced parkinsonism. The clinician can administer the antiparkinsonian drugs orally, and relief should be apparent within hours or days. Recommended dosages are diphenhydramine 25 mg two to four times daily, benztropine 1 to 2 mg twice daily, or trihexyphenidyl 2 to 5 mg twice daily.

Rabbit syndrome, a variant of parkinsonism, causes a perioral tremor (rapid chewing movements). This EPS responds to the antiparkinsonian regimen described for parkinsonism.

Dystonia. Also called acute dystonic reaction, dystonia is one of the most serious and subjectively distressing EPS. The clinical presentation and treatment of dystonia during rapid tranquilization are discussed in Chapter 3, Delirium.

Dystonia is characterized by slurred or dysarthric speech from tongue dystonia, eyes painfully diverted upward (oculogyric crisis), head turned to the side (torticollis) or backward (retrocollis), severe extension (arching) of the back (opisthotonos), and, rarely, laryngospasm from contraction of the muscles of the larynx.

The dystonic patient should immediately be given I.V. antiparkinsonian drugs (such as diphenhydramine 50 mg or benztropine 2 mg). If symptoms persist, the clinician should repeat the dose after 5 minutes. On discharge, the patient should be given a 3-day supply of an oral antiparkinsonian drug (such as diphenhydramine 25 to 50 mg three times daily or benztropine 1 to 2 mg twice daily) and referred to the prescribing physician.

Although dystonia is rarely life-threatening, this syndrome is frightening to the patient and may contribute to subsequent noncompliance with the medication regimen. For patients started on neuroleptic agents in the emergency setting, the clinician must consider prescribing antiparkinsonian drugs to prevent dystonia in those patients being discharged or held for a few days in the crisis area. Although increasing evidence supports this strategy, it may not be needed in every case.

Preventive use of antiparkinsonian drugs concurrently with neuroleptic agents is indicated when the patient:

• has a history of a dystonic reaction.
• is receiving a high-potency antipsychotic agent.
• is given a depot injection.
• is realistically fearful of side effects.
• is paranoid and would interpret the side effect as an assault.

Caution the patient about the potential toxicity of the antiparkinsonian agent and provide instructions about how to deal with future reactions. (The usual response is to return to the emergency service.)

Be alert to the drug abuser who fakes acute dystonia to obtain antiparkinsonian agents for their euphoric properties. Suspect prescription drug abuse in a patient who appears to have dystonia but has not recently been started on a neuroleptic agent or received a depot injection within the past week.

Akathisia. Motor restlessness can occur after the start of antipsychotic drug therapy, after an increase in dosage, or after a depot injection of fluphenazine (Prolixin) or haloperidol decanoate (Haldol). The akathisic patient cannot sit still, which is sometimes described as a "racing motor" inside the patient. This EPS is more common than suspected and is extremely distressing to the patient. Severe akathisia has been associated with self-destructive and homicidal behavior.

The most critical initial intervention is to provide immediate relief, if possible. The medications for EPS, diphenhydramine 50 mg I.M. or benztropine 2 mg I.M., are widely used but sometimes ineffective. Sedatives, such as lorazepam (Ativan) 2 mg orally or 1 mg I.M., may reduce the dysphoria of akathisia for a few hours. The novel approach of using propranolol (Inderal) 20 to 60 mg/day is worth considering for refractory cases of akathisia. However, propranolol is contraindicated in patients with asthma, congestive heart failure, cardiac conduction defects, and diabetes (Neppe, 1989).

The patient with akathisia may feel a loss of control. Reassure the patient that akathisia is a drug side effect, not a worsening of the illness. Brief hospitalization may be beneficial in severe or unresponsive cases.

Tardive dyskinesia. Unique in both its physiology and frequent lack of reversibility, tardive dyskinesia (TD) usually appears after years of neuroleptic treatment as involuntary movements of the mouth or extremities. Because the syndrome can also occur within months of starting neuroleptic therapy, warn all patients receiving such treatment about the possibility of TD. Although not an emergency,

TD can lead to physical and social disability because of the uncontrollable abnormal movements.

No immediate treatment is necessary; the long-term approach to the problem must be worked out between the patient and his prescribing physician. However, the emergency clinician can alert the physician and tell the patient (without alarming him) to discuss the abnormal movements with the psychiatrist.

The physiology of TD renders antiparkinsonian drugs useless; these drugs may even intensify TD symptoms (Mason and Granacher, 1980). If a TD patient is taking antiparkinsonian agents, consider discontinuing this medication.

In every case, document all abnormal movements, both for continuity of care and medicolegal reasons.

Autonomic effects

Antipsychotic drugs have diverse effects, including blockade of cholinergic (muscarinic) and alpha-adrenergic neuroreceptors, both in the CNS and peripherally. As a rule, these effects are more likely to occur with low-potency than high-potency drugs.

Anticholinergic effects. These autonomic side effects include dry mouth, constipation, blurred vision, urinary hesitancy, palpitation, and light-headedness. Many patients respond to a cholinergic agent, such as bethanechol (Urecholine) 25 mg three times daily. Reducing the dosage of the antipsychotic drug or eliminating an antiparkinsonian agent is commonly necessary to relieve these peripheral symptoms.

Central anticholinergic syndrome. Low-potency neuroleptic drugs can also cause CNS toxicity in the form of delirium or central anticholinergic syndrome. Other causes of this syndrome are atropine-like or antiparkinsonian drugs, antidepressants, and over-the-counter medications. In addition to the mental status features of delirium, the clinician should look for the symptoms of central anticholinergic syndrome, which include dry skin, flushed face, dilated and unreactive pupils, tachycardia, diminished or absent bowel sounds, and urine retention.

Begin treatment with physostigmine (Antilirium) 1 to 2 mg I.V. (slow push) or I.M. (Dubin et al., 1986). Because physostigmine's duration of action is only 2 hours, the dose can be repeated in 2-hour intervals, or more frequently if needed. Overly aggressive treatment may precipitate a cholinergic crisis, which can be reversed with atropine 0.5 mg for each 1 mg of physostigmine (Hall et al., 1981). Further complications of physostigmine treatment are vomiting, hypotension, and seizures.

Hypotension. Through alpha-adrenergic blockade, neuroleptic agents — especially chlorpromazine and thioridazine — can lower blood pressure. This effect is most evident when the patient stands or rises after bed rest (orthostatic hypotension). Severe hypotension (systolic blood pressure less than 60 mm Hg) is a medical emergency.

The hypotensive patient who comes to the emergency service should be kept supine in the reverse Trendelenberg position. I.V. fluids should be administered for volume expansion. Begin a pharmacologic intervention with alpha-adrenergic drugs, such as metaraminol (Aramine). Beta-adrenergic agonist drugs, such as isoproterenol (Isuprel), and mixed alpha- and beta-adrenergic drugs should not be used because they can exacerbate the hypotension (Dubin and Feld, 1989).

Neuroleptic malignant syndrome

Neuroleptic malignant syndrome (NMS) has been recognized since neuroleptic agents were first used but has only recently received widespread attention (Lazarus et al., 1989). NMS is a serious, potentially fatal syndrome of muscular rigidity, hyperpyrexia, autonomic instability, and diminished arousal. The pathophysiology of NMS is being studied, with the focus on dopamine neurotransmission (Lazarus et al., 1989).

To be diagnosed with NMS, a patient must concurrently exhibit all five of the diagnostic criteria proposed by Lazarus et al. (1989):
• treatment with neuroleptic agents within 7 days of onset of symptoms (within 4 weeks for depot drugs)
• hyperthermia (greater than or equal to 100.4° F [38° C])
• muscle rigidity
• three of the following: change in mental status, tachycardia, hypertension or hypotension, tachypnea or hypoxia, creatine phos-

phokinase elevation or myoglobinuria, leukocytosis, or metabolic acidosis
• symptoms not caused by systemic or neuropsychiatric illness.

Once NMS is recognized or suspected, the clinician must stop all psychotropic medications, including anticholinergic antiparkinsonian drugs. Initiate life-support measures to reduce the patient's temperature, increase oxygenation, and stabilize the blood pressure and heart rate. Carry out NMS treatment in collaboration with medical specialists.

Pharmacologic intervention to treat the somatic symptoms include (Lazarus et al., 1989):
• dantrolene (Dantrium). This skeletal muscle relaxant may reduce the morbidity associated with rigidity. Dosages are 1 to 10 mg/kg I.V. (single bolus) or 50 to 600 mg/day orally in divided doses.
• dopamine agonists. Bromocriptine (Parlodel), a direct dopamine agonist, can be used alone or in combination with dantrolene. Dosages range from 7.5 to 45 mg three times daily. Other dopamine agonists are amantadine (Symmetrel) and levodopa-carbidopa.
• benzodiazepines. Although these drugs have no direct impact on NMS, they may reduce the patient's agitation. They are a safe alternative to neuroleptic agents, which are contraindicated in patients with NMS.

Other effects

Patients may report the following problems but are not usually aware that these are drug side effects.

Sexual dysfunction. Thioridazine can produce retrograde ("dry") ejaculation. Patients with this complaint can be switched to another neuroleptic agent, such as chlorpromazine. Neuroleptic drugs also can cause lowered libido, amenorrhea, hyperprolactinemia, and galactorrhea (also seen in men).

Sunburn. Patients may show signs of photosensitivity, including severe sunburn and deep pigmentation of the skin after prolonged exposure to the sun. Advise patients receiving neuroleptic medication to avoid the sun as much as possible, to wear protective clothing and hats, and to use a sunblocking lotion.

Heatstroke. Patients on neuroleptic medication may have an impaired ability to dissipate heat. The clinician must differentiate this drug effect on thermoregulation from NMS.

Rash. A rash, especially on the torso, may be caused by neuroleptic agents. Patients with a rash can be given an antihistamine or switched to an antipsychotic agent of a different chemical class.

Blood dyscrasias. Neuroleptic drugs can lower the white blood cell count, which is benign, and cause agranulocytosis (a decrease in neutrophils), which is rare and serious. Early signs of agranulocytosis—persistent sore throat, mouth ulceration, chills, and fever—can be identified in the emergency setting. If a patient has agranulocytosis, immediately discontinue the neuroleptic medication and refer the patient to an internist or hematologist. Blood should be drawn for a "stat" complete blood count and differential.

Drug interactions

Neuroleptic agents used in combination with antidepressants, antianxiety drugs, or anticonvulsants can increase sedation. Antidepressants can also increase anticholinergic and hypotensive effects, while antiparkinsonian agents can increase anticholinergic symptoms and predispose the patient to delirium. Concomitant use of lithium carbonate (Eskalith) may increase the patient's risk for NMS. Other drug interactions include antihypertensive drugs with low-potency neuroleptics, such as chlorpromazine, which can interfere with or potentiate blood pressure effects. Beta blockers can inhibit chlorpromazine metabolism and raise the blood levels of this drug. Levodopa (Dopar) combined with a neuroleptic agent blocks its effect in Parkinson's disease. Phenytoin (Dilantin) metabolism may be reduced, leading to increased phenytoin blood levels and toxicity.

Overdose

An overdose with neuroleptic drugs alone is rarely fatal. However, when tricyclic antidepressants, antiparkinsonian agents, sedatives, or alcohol are combined with a neuroleptic agent, the mortality risk increases. The clinician's immediate concern is to treat the coma, hypothermia, hypotension, and EPS that can result from an overdose. After the patient is medically cleared, the psychiatric condition that caused the patient to take the overdose should be treated in the hospital.

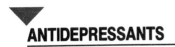

ANTIDEPRESSANTS

Medications used to treat depression are of concern for several reasons. Depressed patients may intentionally overdose themselves. Elderly patients, among whom depression is prevalent, are susceptible to autonomic side effects. Adverse drug reactions that lead to noncompliance expose the patient to increased morbidity from depression, and the drug treatment of depression is typically lengthy, which increases the likelihood that a toxic reaction will develop. The clinician in the psychiatric emergency service is called on to examine patients with various toxic conditions caused by antidepressant drugs.

General effects

Because antidepressant drugs can cause both sedation and arousal, a patient may complain of either somnolence or restlessness. As a rule, tricyclic drugs (amitriptyline [Elavil], nortriptyline, [Aventyl], imipramine [Tofranil], desipramine [Norpramin], trimipramine [Surmontil], and doxepin [Sinequan]) exert their sedative effects in the first few weeks of treatment. Amoxapine [Asendin] and maprotiline [Ludiomil] can also cause sedation within a few weeks of the start of therapy. Trazodone (Desyrel), a sedating nontricyclic antidepressant, can be used to relieve insomnia in a depressed patient.

Antidepressants can cause agitation, restlessness, nervousness, or insomnia. The monoamine oxidase (MAO) inhibitors (phenelzine [Nardil] and tranylcypromine [Parnate]) may trigger an early amphetamine-like effect, including jitteriness and insomnia. Fluoxetine [Prozac] tends to exert its activating effect at about 2 weeks, when its serum level is established. This activating effect can progress to anxiety and agitation. The effect may also be seen with clomipramine (Anafranil) and bupropion (Wellbutrin), drugs that may also reduce seizure threshold.

The clinician can treat general side effects of antidepressant medication by reducing the dosage, prescribing sedating antidepressants to improve the sleep-wake cycle, or switching drugs. Always consult the prescribing physician before beginning any intervention. Giving the patient a new prescription for a benzodiazepine to counteract the effect of an antidepressant is not recommended.

Autonomic effects

The effects of tricyclic drugs on the autonomic nervous system are similar to those produced by low-potency antipsychotic agents and include hypotension (light-headedness upon standing up), blurred vision, sweating, dry mouth, constipation, and urine retention. Of the tricyclic agents, nortriptyline causes the least hypotension. In contrast, MAO inhibitors can significantly lower blood pressure, which is sometimes forgotten because of their more notorious "cheese reaction" (hypertension precipitated by tyramine-containing foods and beverages).

MAO inhibitors and hypertensive crisis. Patients taking the antidepressants phenelzine or tranylcypromine must adhere to food and drug restrictions to prevent a hypertensive crisis. Foods to be avoided are wine and beer, aged cheeses, cured meats, pickled herring, chopped liver, and yeast extracts. Forbidden drugs include stimulants, diet pills, decongestants, local anesthetics containing epinephrine, meperidine (Demerol), opiates, levodopa, and other antidepressants. Patients on MAO inhibitors who report severe headache must be examined for a hypertensive crisis. Any patient who is unfamiliar with the food and drug restrictions should be given a list.

The clinician can treat the hypotensive effect of an antidepressant drug by decreasing the dosage, instituting bedtime dosing, or switching to another agent. Consider adding ephedrine (Ephed II) for hypotension (but not if the patient is taking an MAO inhibitor) or bethanechol for anticholinergic effects. For an MAO inhibitor-induced hypertensive crisis, emergency intervention includes administration of phentolamine (Regitine) 5 mg I.M. or I.V. or other potent antihypertensive agents. Staff members should follow the hospital's code protocols. Outpatients treated with MAO inhibitors are sometimes given a 20-mg capsule of nifedipine (Procardia) to use in case of severe headache, sometimes the first sign of a hypertensive crisis. However, such patients must be cautioned that this self-treatment can lead to hypotension.

Other effects

Because antidepressant drugs have diverse effects, the emergency clinician may encounter patients with some of the following complaints.

Sexual dysfunction. Erectile dysfunction, priapism (with trazodone only), and anorgasmia (especially in women taking MAO inhibitors) can be caused by antidepressant drugs.

Drenching sweat. This effect commonly occurs during sleep or as an excessive reaction to heat.

Tinnitus. Patients may report an uncomfortable ringing or rushing sound in their ears.

Delirium. This side effect is predominantly seen in elderly persons. Amitriptyline and other sedating tricyclic antidepressants can cause central anticholinergic syndrome (see Chapter 14, Geriatric Emergencies).

Seizures. High blood levels of tricyclic antidepressants can lower a patient's seizure threshold. Patients taking maprotiline at doses greater than 200 mg/day are at especially high risk. A combination of a tricyclic antidepressant and fluoxetine, which is not recommended, can elevate the tricyclic antidepressant's serum levels and induce seizures.

Drug interactions

Sedation can be increased when an antidepressant drug is given in combination with neuroleptics, antianxiety agents, or anticonvulsants. The concomitant use of neuroleptics (especially low potency) increases anticholinergic and hypotensive effects and may increase tricyclic antidepressant blood levels. Fluoxetine can raise the blood levels of other drugs, such as tricyclic antidepressants or haloperidol (Haldol), which may lead to toxicity.

Because of uncertain effects on blood pressure, MAO inhibitors should not be used with other antidepressants, stimulants, diet pills, decongestants, disulfiram (Antabuse), alcohol, opiates, or sedatives.

Tricyclic antidepressants, such as amitriptyline, can interfere with the action of antihypertensive agents, and smoking may reduce tricyclic antidepressant blood levels.

Overdose

Depressed patients are treated with some of the most toxic psychotropic drugs. A 1- or 2-week supply (2 g or less) of a tricyclic antidepressant can constitute a lethal overdose. Patients who have overdosed are delirious and hypotensive and have depressed consciousness and severe anticholinergic toxicity. The resulting cardiac arrhythmias and respiratory depression can be fatal and therefore constitute a medical emergency.

Overdose of a tricyclic antidepressant is both common and dangerous (Callaham and Kassel, 1985; Frommer et al., 1987; Stewart, 1979). Although the patient may look deceptively well, the overdose is rapidly fatal (Frommer et al., 1987; Callaham and Kassel, 1985). Be alert for overdose patients who are medically cleared too quickly (Foulke and Albertson, 1987); such patients can die on a psychiatric unit.

An MAO inhibitor overdose is occasionally fatal but more likely to cause delirium, seizures, and hyperthermia (Lazarus et al., 1989). Overdoses of trazodone and fluoxetine usually do not produce fatal outcomes. Although stimulants (amphetamine and methylphenidate) are rarely used to treat depression, their overdose effects include autonomic overactivity, delirium, seizures, and, occasionally, death.

To treat a tricylic antidepressant overdose, start an I.V. line, monitor the patient's heart, and observe the patient closely (Callaham and Kassel, 1985). Additionally, the patient's stomach contents must be evacuated and activated charcoal administered. Initiate advanced interventions, as needed, for depressed consciousness and respiration, hypotension, arrhythmias, cardiac conduction blocks, and seizures. Once the patient is medically stabilized, usually within 24 hours (Frommer et al., 1987), consider transferring him to a psychiatric setting.

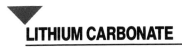

LITHIUM CARBONATE

Lithium carbonate is a remarkably effective medication for preventing episodes of bipolar disorder. However, clinicians and patients alike must know the early signs of toxicity and the importance of regular blood monitoring to maintain safe serum lithium levels.

Toxicity in normal use

Even at ordinary serum levels (0.5 to 1.2 mEq/liter), lithium can cause side effects severe enough to warrant emergency intervention. These include fine tremor; excessive thirst (polydipsia); excessive urination (polyuria); nausea, vomiting, and diarrhea; and mild ataxia. Less serious lithium side effects are acne, dermatitis, nontoxic goiter, and a benign elevation of the white blood cell count. The intervention consists of obtaining a serum lithium level, keeping the patient hydrated, stopping further doses, and informing the prescribing physician.

Drug interactions

Neuroleptic agents, in combination with lithium, may increase the risk of NMS. Thiazide diuretics, such as hydrochlorothiazide (Esidrix), and nonsteroidal anti-inflammatory drugs can decrease lithium excretion and lead to toxicity.

Overdose

At serum lithium levels exceeding 1.5 to 2.0 mEq/liter, toxic symptoms become more dramatic — coarse tremor, ataxia and slurred speech, nystagmus, and severe vomiting. Serum levels of 4.0 mEq/liter or more are potentially fatal.

Lithium overdose is treated by supportive measures, based on the patient's symptoms and serum level. According to Schoonover and Gelenberg (1984), in managing a patient with lithium toxicity, the clinician should:

• evaluate the patient as quickly as possible; a lithium overdose can be fatal

• assess clinical signs and symptoms, serum lithium levels, and electrolyte balance to confirm the diagnosis

• order an electrocardiogram and monitor vital signs

- discontinue the lithium treatment
- support the patient's vital functions and monitor cardiac status
- limit absorption of the drug (If the patient is alert, an emetic is used. If the patient is obtunded, nasogastric suction is used, possibly for several days.)
- prevent infection in comatose patients by body rotation and respiratory therapy
- hydrate the patient vigorously (ideally, 5 to 6 liters/day) and monitor and balance electrolyte levels.

Treating severe lithium intoxication (serum lithium level greater than 4 mEq/liter) is a complex medical intervention, and such issues as forced diuresis and peritoneal dialysis remain controversial (Jefferson et al., 1987). Thus, treatment of a patient with severe lithium intoxication should be left to experienced internists and emergency department physicians.

Educational intervention

All patients should understand the need for regulating the serum level of lithium within a narrow range. In addition, instruct patients to use table salt regularly. However, patients on lithium do not need salt tablets in the summer, since sweating, unlike gross dehydration, does not increase lithium levels.

Patients should know that they can take their total daily dose of lithium at bedtime and that blood for lithium levels must be drawn at the same time relative to the last dose (usually 8 to 12 hours afterward). Patients should have blood tests for kidney and thyroid function twice a year so that any serious change in lithium clearance can be detected early.

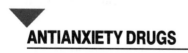

ANTIANXIETY DRUGS

Benzodiazepines, the principal drugs used in the emergency treatment of anxiety, are usually safe when used alone (see Chapter 10, Anxiety). However, when taken in combination with alcohol or other drugs, benzodiazepines can cause unwanted effects that lead to emergency visits.

Behavioral effects

Because benzodiazepines are sedatives, the most prevalent sign of toxicity is drowsiness. Sedation, in turn, can lead to impaired co-ordination and cognitive function. In elderly persons, sedation can contribute to hip fracture from falls (Ray, 1987).

To treat simple benzodiazepine intoxication, reduce the patient's dosage and advise him not to drive or engage in any activity requiring alertness. For intoxication complicated by alcohol use, try to detoxify the patient from both substances. Sometimes a patient experiences wild excitement after taking a benzodiazepine in regular doses, usually after having just started the drug. This paradoxical reaction can produce destructive results, including criminal behavior. Benzodiazepines must be discontinued in such patients.

Interdose breakthrough anxiety

The short elimination half-lives of some benzodiazepines, such as alprazolam (Xanax), oxazepam (Serax), lorazepam, and triazolam (Halcion), can cause significant decreases in serum levels between doses, especially if the medication is used only at bedtime or once or twice a day. In a patient who rapidly metabolizes alprazolam, the functional elimination half-life may be as short as 6 hours. If the patient takes alprazolam at 8 a.m., 3 p.m., and 10 p.m., significant gaps in anxiety coverage can ensue.

Patients with interdose breakthrough anxiety are on an emotional roller coaster. The patient may describe a sudden and intense increase in anxiety, accompanied by a craving for the drug. He may interpret these symptoms as a worsening of the condition, leading to requests for increased doses and, occasionally, to uncontrolled self-medication.

Treatment of breakthrough anxiety is best accomplished by the prescribing physician. The emergency clinician who chooses to initiate treatment should consult with the prescribing physician. One intervention is to change the dosing pattern to every 4 hours, if possible, without altering the total dosage. Another intervention is to switch the patient from the benzodiazepine with the short elimination half-life to one with a long elimination half-life, such as diazepam (Valium), chlordiazepoxide (Librium), or clorazepate (Tranxene).

If the treatment is for chronic anxiety, switching to buspirone may eliminate the breakthrough effect. However, patients must not be switched directly from a benzodiazepine to buspirone, because acute benzodiazepine withdrawal can result.

Withdrawal syndrome

An abstinence syndrome occurs in approximately 40% of patients who withdraw from benzodiazepines after at least 8 months of continuous use (Rickels, 1983). Patients in withdrawal may have a panic attack, insomnia, anxiety, and phobias, or they may become irritable, paranoid, and restless. Somatic symptoms of withdrawal include malaise, tremor, nausea, hyperreflexia, seizures, increased heart rate, and elevated blood pressure. For drugs with short elimination half-life metabolites (alprazolam, lorazepam, oxazepam), the peak risk period for withdrawal occurs 2 to 3 days after the drug is discontinued. Withdrawal symptoms from drugs with long elimination half-life metabolites, such as diazepam, chlordiazepoxide, clorazepate, and flurazepam (Dalmane), are seen within 5 to 7 days. The key clinical discriminator between withdrawal and relapse (a return of symptoms) is that withdrawal symptoms are different from and more intense than the original symptoms.

To treat benzodiazepine withdrawal, the clinician should administer a challenge dose of the drug. If the challenge dose relieves the symptoms within an hour or two, give the patient a prescription for no more than 3 days' worth of the usual dosage. Instruct the patient to visit his prescribing physician as soon as possible.

If the patient is a recognized drug abuser, referral to a detoxification program may be indicated. Do not feel obligated to perpetuate the drug dependency, but treat acute withdrawal symptoms.

Buspirone

A nonsedating antianxiety drug, buspirone (BuSpar) is a partial serotonin agonist that occasionally exacerbates anxiety or insomnia. Many patients overcome this side effect and benefit greatly from buspirone treatment. The usual dosage ranges from 5 mg four times daily to 10 mg three times daily. Buspirone can cause a dysphoric reaction if a large dose (about 40 mg) is given all at once, but the drug does not cause significant overdose toxicity.

Drug interactions

Benzodiazepines increase sedation caused by neuroleptics, antidepressants, anticonvulsants, and alcohol. Buspirone should not be used in patients taking MAO inhibitors because it can induce hypertension. In addition, buspirone may displace digoxin (Lanoxin) from blood proteins, which can cause digoxin toxicity. Antacids can interfere with benzodiazepine absorption and decrease the drug's effect. Smoking can reduce benzodiazepine blood levels.

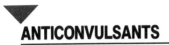

ANTICONVULSANTS

Carbamazepine (Tegretol) is commonly used to treat complex partial seizures (temporal lobe epilepsy) that have a behavioral component, such as aggression, perceptual disturbances, and paranoia. Carbamazepine has also been used in combination with lithium to prevent the mood swings of bipolar disorder.

Toxicity

Toxic doses of carbamazepine can produce slurred speech, ataxia, sedation, and a worsening of seizures. The clinician who suspects toxicity should draw blood for serum level tests. Hematologic disturbances associated with carbamazepine overdose include aplastic anemia (low red blood cell count), agranulocytosis (low white blood cell count), and thrombocytopenia (low platelet count). Patients who complain of fever, sore throat, and malaise may be suffering from carbamazepine-induced agranulocytosis. In such cases, the clinician should draw blood for a "stat" complete blood cell count and differential and consult a medical specialist.

Drug interactions

Using carbamazepine with MAO inhibitors can precipitate a hypertensive crisis. Verapamil (Calan), cimetidine (Tagamet), and propoxyphene (Darvon) increase carbamazepine levels, whereas phenobarbital (Barbita), phenytoin (Dilantin), and primidone (Mysoline) lower them. Carbamazepine itself can lower blood levels of warfarin (Coumadin), phenytoin, haloperidol, and theophylline (TheoDur).

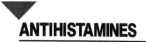

ANTIHISTAMINES

Antihistaminic agents, such as diphenhydramine (Benadryl) and hydroxyzine (Atarax), are an alternative to benzodiazepines and can be used as bedtime or as-needed sedatives. Despite their reputation as benign drugs, antihistamines can cause significant toxic effects, including delirium, seizures, respiratory arrest, and death. Drug abusers may attempt to snort or inject powdered forms of antihistamines.

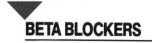

BETA BLOCKERS

Patients treated with propranolol (Inderal) or atenolol (Tenormin) for situational anxiety (test taking, stage fright) or as an adjunct in panic disorder may complain of depression, lethargy, insomnia, nightmares, and sexual dysfunction. Serious toxicity causes hypotension or bradycardia.

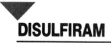

DISULFIRAM

Disulfiram (Antabuse) is an adjunctive therapy for maintaining abstinence in alcoholic patients. By blocking the liver enzyme aldehyde dehydrogenase, disulfiram causes faulty alcohol metabolism, which leads to an accumulation of acetaldehyde. This, in turn, produces various noxious symptoms, such as severe, throbbing headache; nausea; vomiting; chest pain and palpitations; hypotension; fainting; anxiety; hyperventilation; weakness; sweating; and thirst (*Springhouse Drug Reference,* 1988). Severe reactions include cardiovascular collapse, seizures, and death. In addition to the reaction with alcohol, disulfiram has a side effect profile that includes sedation, fatigue, delirium, depression, psychosis, and headache. Brief treatment with a neuroleptic agent may be indicated in disulfiram-induced psychosis or delirium. Otherwise, discontinuation of the drug and outpatient follow-up are sufficient. The clinician must warn patients who discontinue disulfiram that the reaction with alcohol can persist for several days or more.

REFERENCES

Baldessarini, R.J. *Chemotherapy in Psychiatry.* Boston: Harvard University Press, 1985.

Callaham, M., and Kassel, D. "Epidemiology of Fatal Tricyclic Antidepressant Ingestion: Implications for Management," *Annals of Emergency Medicine* 14(1):1-9, January 1985.

Dubin, W.R., Weiss, K.J., and Dorn, J.M. "Pharmacotherapy of Psychiatric Emergencies," *Journal of Clinical Psychopharmacology* 6(4):210-222, August 1986.

Dubin, W.R., and Feld, J.A. "Rapid Tranquilization of the Violent Patient," *American Journal of Emergency Medicine* 7(3):313-320, May 1989.

Foulke, G.E., and Albertson, T.E. "QRS Interval in Tricyclic Antidepressant Overdosage: Inaccuracy as a Toxicity Indicator in Emergency Settings," *Annals of Emergency Medicine* 16(2):160-163, February 1987.

Frommer, D.A., et al. "Tricyclic Antidepressant Overdose: A Review," *JAMA* 257(4):521-526, January 23, 1987.

Hall, R.C.W., Feinsilver, D.L., and Holt, R.E. "Anticholinergic Psychosis: Differential Diagnosis and Management," *Psychosomatics* 22(7):581-587, July 1981.

Jefferson, J.W., et al. *Lithium Encyclopedia for Clinical Practice,* 2nd ed. Washington, D.C.: American Psychiatric Press, 1987.

Lazarus, A., et al. *The Neuroleptic Malignant Syndrome and Related Conditions.* Washington, D.C.: American Psychiatric Press, 1989.

Mason, A.S., and Granacher, R.P. *Clinical Handbook of Antipsychotic Drug Therapy.* New York: Bruner/Mazel, 1980.

Neppe, V. *Innovative Psychopharmacotherapy.* New York: Raven Press, 1989.

Ray, W.A., et al. "Psychotropic Drug Use and Risk of Hip Fracture," *New England Journal of Medicine* 316(7):363-369, February 12, 1987.

Rickels, K., et al. "Long-Term Diazepam Therapy and Clinical Outcome," *JAMA* 250(6):767-771, August 12, 1983.

Schoonover, S.C., and Gelenberg, A.J. "Emergency Presentations Related to Psychiatric Medication," in *Emergency Psychiatry: Concepts, Methods, and Practices.* Edited by Bassuk, E.L., and Birk, A.W. New York: Plenum Press, 1984.

Springhouse Drug Reference. Springhouse, Pa.: Springhouse Corporation, 1988.

Stewart, R.D. "Tricyclic Antidepressant Poisoning," *American Family Physician* 19(5):136-144, May 1979.

APPENDIX A

SIGNS AND SYMPTOMS OF MAJOR PSYCHIATRIC SYNDROMES

SYNDROME	BEHAVIOR	SPEECH	THOUGHT PROCESS	THOUGHT CONTENT
Delirium	Agitation (occasionally quiet), carphologia	Nonspecific	Tangentiality, incoherence	Variable; delusions
Dementia	Apathy, apraxia, echopraxia	Echolalia, aphasia	Perseveration	Variable; few if any delusions
Schizophrenia	Social withdrawal, agitation	Rambling, mutism	Loose associations, blocking	Bizarre, persecutory delusions, ideas of reference
Mania	Hyperactivity, gregariousness	Rapid, forceful	Flight of ideas	Delusions of grandeur, paranoia
Depression	Motor retardation, occasional agitation	Lack of spontaneity, slow pace and monotonous tone	Paucity of thought	Helplessness, hopelessness, delusions of guilt, self-reproach, poverty, somatic delusions

Source: Dubin, W.R., and Weiss, K.J., "Emergency Psychiatry," in *Psychiatry,* vol. 2. Edited by Cavenar, J.O. Philadelphia: J.B. Lippincott Co., 1989. Adapted with permission of the publisher.

PERCEP-TION	AFFECT	ORIENTATION AND MEMORY	ONSET AND DURATION	PHYSICAL FINDINGS
Illusions, hallucinations (especially visual)	Fear, anxiety	Disorientation, memory impairment, clouded consciousness	Acute (hours to days), with fluctuating symptoms	Abnormal vital signs
Few if any hallucinations	Lability	Disorientation, memory impairment	Insidious	Frontal lobe release signs (such as grasp reflex)
Hallucinations (usually auditory)	Blunted, flat, inappropriate affect	Intact	Symptoms for 6 months	None
Hallucinations possible	Elation, frequent irritability	Intact	Symptoms for 1 week	None
Few if any hallucinations	Depression, sadness, despondence	Intact	Symptoms for 2 weeks	None

APPENDIX B

DIAGNOSING PSYCHOSIS

SYNDROME	HISTORY
Delirium (Consult Chapter 3)	• Acute onset (hours to days) • Diagnosed medical illness • Currently taking medications for medical illness • Over age 40 and no previous psychiatric history
Drug and alcohol intoxication and withdrawal (Consult Chapters 4 and 5)	• Acute onset (hours to days) • Previous history of treatment for drugs or alcohol
Schizophrenia (Consult Chapter 6)	• History of schizophrenia
Mania (Consult Chapter 6)	• History of mania and depression
Depression (Consult Chapter 9)	• History of depression or mania • Recent personal loss • Sleep disturbance • Loss of appetite • Loss of sex drive

MENTAL STATUS	PHYSICAL FINDINGS
• Stupor or lethargy • Illusions • Visual hallucinations • Disorientation • Memory impairment • Sundowner's syndrome • Impaired attention span • Fluctuating symptoms	• High blood pressure • Sweating • Rapid pulse • Rapid breathing
• Stupor and lethargy or agitation • Visual hallucinations • Tactile hallucinations • Delusions	• Alcohol odor on breath • Needle tracks on arms • Nasal septum erosion • Ataxia • Slurred speech • Hyperreflexia • Pupillary changes • High blood pressure • Sweating • Rapid pulse • Rapid breathing
• Delusions • Hallucinations (usually auditory) • Disorganized, incoherent thinking • Flat or inappropriate affect	• Poor hygiene
• Elevated, expansive, or irritable mood • Hyperactivity • Flight of ideas • Rapid, forceful speech • Decreased need for sleep	• Hoarse voice
• Somatic delusions • Delusions of guilt • Self-reproach • Suicidal ideation • Hopelessness	• Weight loss • Physical debilitation

APPENDIX C

FOLSTEIN MINI-MENTAL STATE EXAMINATION

The Folstein Mini-Mental State Examination is the preferred tool for assessing the mental status of a patient with suspected cognitive impairment. To perform the examination, ask the patient to follow a series of simple commands that test his ability to understand and perform cognitive functions. Award a designated point value for successful completion of each instruction, then total the scores to determine the patient's mental status. Scores of 26 to 30 indicate that the patient is normal; 22 to 25, mildly impaired; and less than 22, significantly impaired.

PATIENT INSTRUCTIONS	MAXIMUM SCORE	ACTUAL SCORE
Orientation		
• Ask the patient to name the year, season, date, day, and month. (Score one point for each correct response.)	5	( )
• Ask the patient to name his state, city, street, and house address, and the room in which he is standing. (Score one point for each correct response.)	5	( )
Comprehension		
Name three objects, pausing 1 second between each name. Then ask the patient to repeat all three names. (Score one point for each correct response.) Repeat this exercise until the patient can correctly name all three objects (the patient will be tested on his ability to recall this information later in the examination).	3	( )
Attention and calculation		
Ask the patient to count backward by sevens, beginning at 100; have him stop after counting out five numbers. Alternatively, ask the patient to spell "World" backward. (Score one point for each correct response.)	5	( )
Recall		
Ask the patient to restate the name of the three objects previously identified in the examination. (Score one point for each correct response.)	3	( )

FOLSTEIN MINI-MENTAL STATE EXAMINATION (continued)

PATIENT INSTRUCTIONS	MAXIMUM SCORE	ACTUAL SCORE
Language		
• Point to a pencil and a watch. Ask the patient to identify each object. (Score one point for each correct response.)	2	( )
• Ask the patient to repeat "No ifs, ands, or buts." (Score one point for a correct response.)	1	( )
• Ask the patient to take a paper in his right hand, then fold the paper in half, then put the paper on the floor. (Score one point for each correct response to this three-part command.)	3	( )
• Ask the patient to read and obey the written instruction "Close your eyes." (Score one point for a correct response.)	1	( )
• Ask the patient to write a sentence. (Score one point for a correct response.)	1	( )
• Ask the patient to copy the following design. (Score one point for a correct response.)	1	( )

Adapted with permission from Folstein, M.F., et al. "Mini-Mental State: A Practical Method for Grading the Cognitive State of Patients for the Clinician," *Journal of Psychiatric Research* 12:196-97, 1975.

APPENDIX D

GLOSSARY OF STREET DRUG NAMES

STIMULANTS*

Bennies
Blue angels
Chris
Christine
Christmas trees
Coast to coast
Coke (cocaine)
Copilot
Crisscross
Crossroads
Crystal (I.V. metham-
  phetamine)†
Dexies

Double cross
Flake (cocaine)
Footballs
Glass (methamphet-
  amine)
Gold dust (cocaine)
Green and clears
Hearts
Ice (methamphet-
  amine)
Lip poppers
Meth
Oranges

Peaches
Pep pills
Pinks
Roses
Snow (cocaine)
Speed
Speedball (heroin plus
  cocaine)
Truck drivers
Uppers
Ups
Wake-ups
Whites

PHENCYCLIDINE (PCP)

Angel dust
Aurora
Bust bee
Cheap cocaine
Cosmos
Criptal
Dummy mist
Goon
Green
Guerrilla

Hot
Jet
K
Lovely
Mauve
Mist
Mumm dust
Peace pill
Purple
Rocket fuel

Shermans
Sherms
Special L.A. coke
Superacid
Supercoke
Supergrass
Superjoint
Tranq
Whack

ANALGESICS

Heroin

Brown
H
H and stuff

Horse
Junk
Scat

Shit
Skag
Smack

Other

Black (opium)
Blue velvet (paregoric
  plus amphetamine)
Dollies (methadone)†
M (morphine)

Microdots (morphine)
PG or PO (paregoric)
Pinks and grays (pro-
  poxyphene hydro-
  chloride)

Poppy (opium)
Tar (opium)
Terp (terpin hydrate or
  cough syrup with co-
  deine)

GLOSSARY OF STREET DRUG NAMES (continued)

CNS DEPRESSANTS**

Blue birds	Green and whites	Seccy
Blue devil	(chlordiazepoxide)	Seggy
Blue heaven	Greenies	Sleepers
Blues	Nembies	T-birds
Bullets	Peanuts	Toolies
Dolls†	Peter (chloral hydrate)	Tranqs
Double trouble	Rainbows	Yellow jackets
Downs	Red devils	Yellows
Goofballs	Roaches (chlordiaz-	
	epoxide)†	

HALLUCINOGENS

Acid (LSD)	Crystal†	Mescal (mescaline)
Blue dots (LSD)	Cube (LSD)	Owsleys (LSD)
Cactus (mescaline)	D (LSD)	Pearly gates (morning
		glory seeds)

CANNABINOLS

Acapulco gold	Jive	Roach†
Bhang	Joint	Rope
Brick	Key or kee	Sativa
Charas	Lid	Stick
Gage	Locoweed	Sweet Lucy
Ganja	Mary Jane	Tea
Grass	MJ	Texas tea
Hash	Muggles	Weed
Hay	Pot	Yesca
Hemp	Reefer	

SOLVENTS AND INHALANTS

Huffing	Locker room	Snappers
Jac aroma	Poppers	Sniffers
Kicks	Rush	

* A form of amphetamine unless otherwise stated.

† Many drugs have the same name.

**Moderate length of action like secobarbital unless otherwise noted.

Source: Schuckit, M.A. *Drug and Alcohol Abuse,* 3rd ed. New York: Plenum Publishing Corp., 1989. Reprinted with permission of the publisher.

INDEX

t refers to a table

t refers to a table

D

t refers to a table

Spouse abuse – *continued*
  mental status findings in, 176
  physical findings in, 176
Stelazine. *See* Trifluoperazine.
Stimulant abuse, 55-61
  differential diagnosis in, 57-58
  disposition of patient with, 59-60
  educational intervention in, 59
  interpersonal intervention in, 58
  laboratory studies in, 56-57
  medicolegal considerations in, 60-61
  mental status findings in, 55
  pharmacologic intervention in, 58, 119t
  physical findings in, 55-56
  triage approach to, 56t
  violent behavior in, 119t
Street drug names, glossary of, 280-281t
Suicidal behavior in children and adoles-
      cents, 195-200
  differential diagnosis in, 197-198
  disposition of patient with, 199-200
  educational intervention in, 199
  family assessment in, 197
  interpersonal intervention in, 198
  medicolegal considerations in, 200
  mental status findings in, 196
  pharmacologic intervention in, 199
  physical findings in, 196-197
Suicidal thoughts, 8
Suicide gesture, 128, 133, 197
Suicide risk
  clinical indicators of, 131t
  evaluation of, 130-133
Sundowner's syndrome, 25
Supplements for alcohol withdrawal, 44, 46
Survivors, grieving, 151-153
  concluding meetings with, 153
  initial interventions with, 151
  organ donation and, 152-153
  reactions of, 152
  viewing of body by, 152

T

Talbutal, 76t
Tangentiality, 7
Tardive dyskinesia, 258-259
Tegretol, 271
Telephone callers, abusive
  intervention with, 245
  self-destructive behavior in, 136
Temazepam
  duration of action, 76t
  for generalized anxiety disorder, 164
  phenobarbital withdrawal conversion from,
      79t
Tenormin, 272
Therapeutic relationship, development of,
      133-134
Thiamine
  for alcohol amnestic disorder, 49
  for alcohol withdrawal syndrome, 46
Thioridazine, 261
  for akinesia, 256
  for borderline personality disorder, 247
  for stimulant abuse, 58
Thiothixene
  for alcohol hallucinosis, 51
  in alcohol intoxication, 38
  for alcohol withdrawal syndrome, 46
  for delirium, 222
  for dementia, 218
  for depression, 147
  dose for rapid tranquilization, 31t
  for phencyclidine abuse, 63
  for self-destructive behavior, 137
  for stimulant abuse, 58
  for violent patient, 119t
Thorazine. *See* Chlorpromazine.
Transitory euphoria, 164
Tranxene. *See* Clorazepate.
Treatment refusal, violent patient and, 124
Triazolam, 76t
Tricyclic antidepressants, 263-266
  effects, 264-265
  interactions and, 265-266
  overdose, 266

t refers to a table